SELF-CARE R...

5 Pi...
...t
Prevent Burnout
and
Build Sustainable Resilience
for
Helping Professionals

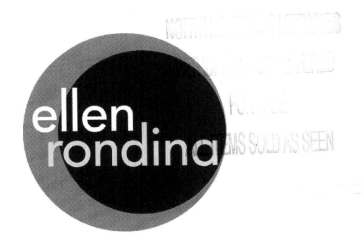

ELLEN RONDINA
Find Your Rhythm

Copyright © 2018 Ellen Rondina

All rights reserved. No part of this book may be reproduced in any form or by any electronic or mechanical means, including information storage and retrieval systems, without permission in writing from the publisher, except by reviewers, who may quote brief passages in a review.

ISBN: 978-1-983-03343-8
Editor: Nina Shoroplova
Proofreader: Rebecca Coates
Cover design: Angie Alaya
Printed in the United States of America
Published by ellen rondina
ellen@ellenrondina.com
Upland, CA 91786
Visit www.ellenrondina.com

PRAISE FOR
SELF-CARE REVOLUTION

"The Self-Care Revolution has arrived! Self-care is a practical, person-centered set of activities that we should all be doing to maintain our health, wellness, and wellbeing. Through self-care people can be healthier and remain so into old age, managing minor ailments themselves. They can also better manage, delay, or even prevent the appearance of lifestyle diseases such as heart attacks, strokes, diabetes, and many cancers.

"Playing a vital role in health and not least in encouraging people to self-care, helping professionals are in the front line of the revolution. They can and should be role models themselves, practising what they preach. In her valuable eBook, Ellen Rondina focuses on helping the care-giving professionals themselves to self-care. The book presents a practical guide to what self-care is, assessing one's self-care situation, identifying strengths, overcoming barriers, and making a personal self-care plan. Ellen is to be congratulated on this contribution to the self-care revolution."
David E. Webber PhD, President, International Self-Care Foundation (ISF)

"*Self-Care Revolution* is a saving grace to the caregivers and healers of the world that must, in order to continue their much-needed work, take care of themselves first. Ellen's five pillars provide a road map for wellness from the inside out. Combining engaging stories with practical action-oriented steps and journaling exercises, this book will inspire you to live a happier, healthier life."
Kathryn Kemp Guylay, award-winning and bestselling author of six books and transformational leader

"Intelligent... Relevant... and Practical!
"Ellen skillfully leads us on a journey of Self-Evaluation, mindfully highlighting the conflicts faced by caring people working in

demanding and pressured environments. This book is packed with personal and professional insight, which combined with a pragmatic hands-on approach offers the reader a pathway to establish a baseline of real and lasting Self-Care. The workbook is a fabulous Bonus!

"An absolute must for anyone working in the helping professions."

Jenny Florence, Accredited Counsellor, BACP, UKRC. #1 Bestselling author of *7 Steps to Spiritual Empathy* **and** *Mindfulness Meets Emotional Awareness.*

"This is the book I wish I'd had at the beginning of my career as a clinical psychologist! Combining relatable personal examples with her decades of professional experience, Ellen offers practical insights and strategies to deal with the stress and burnout that too often goes hand-in-hand with being a helping professional. She dives deep into self-care practices, going beyond bubble baths and the common things we think about with self-care. Ultimately, she offers a way to relate more compassionately with ourselves, which leads to more resilience for us and better outcomes for those we serve."

Barbara Markway, PhD, Psychologist and Author

"There is no doubt in my mind that Ellen Rondina's new e-book *Self Care Revolution* will become an important tool for first responders and professionals offering trauma informed care. She offers all helping professionals a clear and in-depth way to explore their own self-care needs by identifying five pillars of self-care. Rondina makes it clear that we as providers are responsible for doing this work; however, her book provides us with an organized and thorough road map. The workbook style affords the professional the opportunity to explore their truth, their values, and their obstacles. It is brilliantly written and deeply satisfying and supportive for those who give so much of themselves to their community."

Ann C. Bliss, LCMHC, Private Practice, Owner and Director of the Center for Trauma Intervention

Contents

Acknowledgements 9

Introduction 10
    A Commitment to Ourselves 10
    How This Book Came About 12
    What You'll Find in This Book 13

The Problem 15
    On the Front Lines 15
    Ignoring Self-Care 17
    Compounding Stressors 18
    An Ethical and Spiritual Path 19
    Conclusion 22

The Pillars 23
    Self-Care as an Act of Justice 23
    Conclusion 25

Pillar 1: Define Self-Care 26
    Pillar 1: Define Self-Care — Initial Assessment 26
    Self-Care Is Cultural and Personal 27
    My Self-Care and Self-Management 27
    Other Formal Definitions of Self-Care 31
    Self-Care as Social Justice 33
    Pillar 1: Define Self-Care — Post-Assessment 35
    Conclusion 36

Pillar 2: Write a Values Statement 37
What Is Your "Why"? 37
Pillar 2: Write a Values Statement — Initial Assessment.............. 38
Self-Care Equation 40
Pillar 2: Write a Values Statement — Post-Assessment 44
Conclusion.. 45

Pillar 3: Make a Self-Care Plan 46
Pillar 3: Make a Self-Care Plan — Initial Assessment 47
Example Plans... 47
Organizations' Self-Care Plans 49
Focus on Your Strengths 50
Identify Barriers 51
Take the Time to Prioritize 54
Where Are We Now?.. 56
Pillar 3 Making a Self-Care Plan — Post-Assessment 56
Conclusion.. 57

Pillar 4: Recognize Impairment.. 58
Pillar 4: Recognize Impairment — Initial Assessment.................. 58
Definitions.. 59
Pillar 4: Recognize Impairment — Post-Assessment 64
Conclusion.. 65

Pillar 5: Support Others in Their Self-Care Plans...... 66
Pillar 5 Support Others — Initial Assessment 67
Accountability... 67
Work Environment.. 69
Pillar 5 Support Others — Post-Assessment................................. 73
Conclusion.. 74

Final Thoughts **76**

SELF-CARE REVOLUTION WORKBOOK **79**
    Pillar 1: Define Self-Care..80
    Pillar 2: Write a Values Statement..................................82
    Pillar 3: Make a Self-Care Plan 85
    Pillar 4: Recognize Impairment 94
    Pillar 5: Support Others in Their Self-Care Plans...........96

Sources and Additional Resources **99**

Author Biography **105**

Congratulations! **106**

Acknowledgements

I have been writing books for at least 15 years, if not more. They are in notebooks and journals, and some are sketched out more than others. This was not the book I thought I would publish first, but time and circumstances have brought this to fruition.

I thank the following people:

Kathryn Kemp Guylay and Carol Kline for getting me officially started on my author journey with their course Making Publishing Fun: Get Your Transformational Book Done.

Geoff Affleck and his eBook Bestseller Bootcamp, as I had not even seen or read an eBook before I enrolled in his program.

Nina Shoroplova, author & book editor, for seeing me through the transformational process of editing.

Through Kathryn, Carol, Geoff, and Nina, I was lovingly and expertly guided through a world I knew nothing about: publishing, authorship, online entrepreneurship, and editing.

Kathy Oaks, my "accountabili-buddy," for her weekly support as part of Geoff's eBook Bestseller Bootcamp.

All the amazing professionals who were willing to contribute their own personal stories of struggle and resilience to make this book especially meaningful. All names were changed to protect privacy.

My husband, for his unflinching and total support, which is a gift beyond measure.

My son, for his (sometimes) patient ability to share me with my work, when all he wants to do is come into my office and play flutes or sit on my lap at the computer to press all the keys on my keyboard and play with the mouse.

INTRODUCTION

Love is a combination of care, commitment, knowledge, responsibility, respect and trust.
bell hooks, author

Say YES to YOU. Fall in Love with yourself and embrace your power.

A Commitment to Ourselves
I believe that our society is teetering on the brink between wellness and dis-ease. And unless we caregiving professionals learn how to take care of ourselves, things are not going to get better. But my Revolutionary Self-Care program is designed to do exactly that: make things better — for all of us!

This book is a guide to five important Pillars of establishing a foundation for Self-Care as a permanent and important part of your everyday life and work. For all social workers, teachers, mental health professionals, health care providers, first responders, clergy, coaches, leaders supporting others, and all who identify as a helping professional, this book is for you!

To practice Self-Care is to intentionally engage in activities that help you to be well in any number of areas in your life. I believe this is what is needed right now.

I want you to be resilient — and to be a leader in resilience. I want you to easily and confidently walk the Self-Care talk. I want you to thrive, despite your immersion in a sometimes violent and almost always stressful work environment. I want you to embrace Self-Care as an act of justice.

In many ways, our lives and cultures are fear-based. We are often trying to one-up each other in our efforts, our successes, our busyness. We often struggle to stay young and look young in a culture that doesn't support or honor the aging process. We are surrounded by a culture that says what we have and who we are is never enough.

If those of us who are educated professionals in helping fields feel all of these pressures and stresses, how do the people and communities we are trying to support feel? We need more compassion for ourselves, and we need to offer and show more compassion to our colleagues, who are also living this life of service. I believe that part of our responsibility as helping professionals is to be role models. If we are helping people to be well in any or all aspects of their lives and we are not walking the wellness talk, it will be extremely difficult to ask our clients to make changes toward their own wellness, especially sustainable and meaningful changes.

What we are doing now to care for ourselves is often not enough. Too many of us are not feeling well enough to do our jobs ethically, effectively, and with energy and love. We aren't taking care of our needs and those of our friends and families enough to feel balanced and healthy in our lives. Yet our professional codes demand that we practice Self-Care.

Some of us learn about Self-Care and are asked to practice it as part of our formal education. There are many great books on Self-Care techniques. Yet none of this seems to be translating to us practicing sustained and sustainable Self-Care. So many things vie for our attention and cause us fear. There are so many needs and so many people in crisis. It is time to turn inward and turn toward each other. It is time to mindfully embrace Self-Care as a necessary revolution.

What I see now is too much suffering because of a lack of Self-Care. No matter what is happening in our world, our country, we can weather the storm and still be grounded. We can learn our life's lessons and give of our gifts, talents, and contributions — but only if we are well, taking care of ourselves, taking care of each other, and helping others to be well. Too often and too easily we turn away from each other and from what grounds us. Our systems are failing us when it comes to care and wellness. I see the health care system, our work and employment systems, education systems, and our financial systems as systems that are unwell. These systems seem to be benefitting from poor individual Self-Care. People take out more loans and accumulate more credit card debt than they can handle. This benefits the financial systems but not the individuals. People aren't exercising enough or eating as well as they could, and this keeps the health care industry and pharmaceutical companies hopping, while individuals remain stuck in a cycle of being unwell. Employers are keeping people in golden handcuffs, offering incentives and benefits — like flexibility or the promise of promotion — that feel like they can't be turned down even if the work environment is toxic and unsupportive. This is why embracing Self-Care and focusing on these five Pillars is a Revolutionary act.

We have to be the ones to step up and do better and be better, and those of us who are already doing the work in the field of care, wellness, and service need to be the leaders. We are the ones, and remember, you can be a leader even without any followers.

How This Book Came About
I have been on my own path of Self-Care, wellness, and healing for more than thirty years, following an early childhood with a mix of wonderful love and opportunities and also significant stress and trauma.

In response to this environment, I spent a lot of time thinking about these two opposing experiences coexisting and what it meant. I thought a lot about relationships and human behavior and wellness and spirituality and what I believed about it all. I also ruminated on social justice issues like poverty, violence, and disease, and why people might experience these. I spent hours lying in bed as a child thinking about these concepts and acting them out by myself, taking on different roles and creating new possibilities.

I had nightmares that made me scared and tired, and I decided I would need to change this by learning to control my dreams. I practiced lucid dreaming and was able to actively change what was happening in my nightmares and, therefore, change the narrative and experience I was having. This translated into my waking life as well and empowered me.

I didn't know through all of this that I was practicing Self-Care, but that's what it was.

I also got sick both physically and emotionally and began a biofeedback and guided imagery program at the age of sixteen, after being diagnosed with infectious mononucleosis, chronic fatigue immune dysfunction syndrome, fibromyalgia, and depression. This was my first experience with meditation and learning to mindfully be aware of my body and my body's response to my mind. I started going to acupuncture three times a week and was taking herbs and learning more about a natural way of healing.

My very early path of search and discovery eventually led me to a master's degree in social work, a professional coaching certificate, a ministerial degree, and expertise in several healing modalities. I have worked in universities, private schools, nonprofit organizations, public schools, and with my own business, and all of my life's work and my formal education has a foundation of wellness and Self-Care. My portfolio of teaching and coaching is broad-ranging. It includes music, human behavior, therapeutic modalities, community organizing and change, diversity and inclusivity, parenting, nutrition, stress management, change and growth, mindfulness, meditation, and Self-Care itself. My social work code of ethics requires me to practice Self-Care. My social work, teaching, and coaching require me to be a leader and a model. I believe this path of wellness and Self-Care and love is one of the most important and foundational directions we can walk to change the course of fear and violence we are on right now.

As an author, I am not sharing the intimate details of my path but rather my "why." I share some personal stories in this book, but more importantly, I share my values. I am human and I am fallible. I am also completely committed — a thousand percent — to this path of Self-Care for myself and for you.

What You'll Find in This Book

Throughout this book, you'll see references to two tools we'll be using: your Self-Care baseline, which is an online assessment tool you can find through my website, www.ellenrondina.com, and the Self-Care Revolution workbook that can be found right here as the second part of this manuscript. Please note that after careful consideration, I decided to capitalize Self-Care throughout the book to emphasize the signature importance of it in and for our lives.

Start by taking my Self-Care assessment to establish your Self-Care baseline. You can find it at www.ellenrondina.com/self-care. Take a few minutes now to take the assessment. You will receive a response in your email inbox with your results and some information about what those results might mean. This will give you a baseline of how you are doing with your own Self-Care and, if you date your baseline assessment, you'll be able to refer to it and watch your progress.

In the workbook, I will invite you to complete an initial assessment of each of the five Self-Care Pillars, and subsequently you will be invited to complete a post-assessment. Part of this work being "revolutionary" is the action that you will take. That action starts with the Self-Care Revolution workbook!

Now let's get started!

ONE

THE PROBLEM

Stress is the trash of modern life — we all generate it, but if you don't dispose of it properly, it will pile up and overtake your life.
Danzae Pace, author

On the Front Lines
To practice Self-Care is to intentionally engage in activities that help you to be well in any number of areas in your life. If we are practicing Self-Care, we can feel balanced, energized, centered, grounded, and ready to be of service in our work and in our lives.

In a time of increased violence, fear, and anxiety, and a time of ever-dwindling resources for the people and places who need them the most, the work of teachers, social workers, mental health and other health providers, clergy, first responders, coaches, healers, activists, and others on the front lines is getting so much harder. Our work stressors and demands and the lack of focus and support around Self-Care have made it difficult for helping professionals to practice Self-Care in any kind of sustained and meaningful way. We are working longer hours, we have more clients, we are faced with an increased need from our aging population and from a growing opioid addiction epidemic, and school shootings are in the daily news, just to name a few tangible stresses. Helping professionals are on the front lines of the escalating violence, threats, and unhealthy responsive behaviors, both personally and professionally. This is all happening in our work environments; meanwhile, we try to balance our work's expectations with our own lives, our families, friends, hobbies, and of course, our health and wellness.

Here is the discomfort that Ashley, a mid-career master's-level child protective worker, is currently experiencing:

> *I feel obligated to this particular path because this is what I do. I don't know what else I would do that would feel as important. I love investigations, but I have an indefinable need for something to be different. I'm not sure if this is the job or, if something else changed in my life, whether the job could stay the same? I move faster from being compassionate to being authoritative. I don't know whether this is a red flag for compassion fatigue, or if I am getting better at my job.*

Her experience — she calls it "compassion fatigue" — is unfortunately not unique, and I am certain many of you reading this book can relate. Statistics show how hard and long we work, and the effects of these behaviors and schedules are profound and widespread. We are working longer hours and working during hours of the day when we might otherwise be resting or sleeping. The balance is off, creating a cycle of struggle between our wellness and how we are able to be present and available in our work and in our lives.

> *In July* [2017], *a survey conducted by the National Safety Council found that 97 percent of Americans have at least one of the leading risk factors for fatigue, which include working at night or in the early morning, working long shifts without breaks and working more than 50 hours per week. Forty-three percent of respondents said they do not get enough sleep to think clearly at work, make informed decisions and be productive.* (Bill Ervolino, NorthJersey.com)

Our access to 24/7 media is also taking its toll. Everyone is in the spotlight and pointing fingers; accusations fly all too easily. We continue, as a culture, to honor *busyness* above wellness and balance and, although some form of Self-Care is required in all these professions, it is not usually taken as seriously as it needs to be, and not honored in the same way that busyness, production, and growth are revered.

Ignoring Self-Care
We think about Self-Care from a distance, as something we are supposed to do, and we know it's important, but we haven't really thought about it or made any kind of plan for it. So there is no context or structure or accountability, because there is little foundation or understanding of what Self-Care can be. We are always one-upping each other when it comes to how much we have going on and how much we have to do. It is a badge of honor to be checking and responding to email, stroking our egos to think that we are so important and indispensable. This is especially true for helping professionals, who often feel they need to be superhuman, and they are also often seen as superhuman, feeding the notion that they should not need to ask for help. This all comes at the risk of losing our footing. Often people realize they haven't been taking care of themselves for so long that now it actually might be too late; some realize that, at the least, they might have otherwise avoided some major health problems if they had been practicing Self-Care.

Janis is coming to the end of her helping career and is at the point where she is really reflecting on her path, her different jobs, her Self-Care — or lack thereof — and all of the implications. As the executive director of a battered women's program with very few staff, she was always on call.

> *In addition to the contract work, grant writing, and administration, I also worked in the shelter and provided support there and in court to battered women. It was an incredible job, but with extremely limited resources.*

This was a setup for burnout, and Janis did just that. She was unable to sleep and came to realize that she had experienced vicarious trauma through the stories of her clients. Unfortunately, her next job was also doing emergency on-call work, and during this time she was diagnosed with Stage 1 breast cancer and underwent extensive surgery and chemotherapy. Here's the kicker: even though she took medical leave, she felt guilty for not working. This is also not an uncommon story for helping professionals who have chosen this life of service to others.

> *During the last year there, one of our clients set herself on fire and another killed herself. I realized I was not only sleep deprived, but also emotionally drained. I decided that I would not do any more 24/7 work. I do worry that ignoring my health and working very stressful jobs may have affected my immune system's ability to combat cancer, which I have had twice now.*

The work that Janis was called and compelled to do was extremely exhausting and traumatic, and in fact much of the work we do as helping professionals fits this same picture. The ramifications if we are not caring for ourselves first are potentially fatal. That does not appear to be an exaggeration if you were to ask Janis.

Compounding Stressors
There is corroborating evidence that our stress, secondary trauma, compassion fatigue, and burnout stem from both our perspective of what's happening in the United States, and much of the world, and how that perspective manifests within our work and work environments.

The American Psychological Association released the first phase of its current "Stress in America" report (conducted in August 2017) on November 1, 2017. There are some seriously concerning statistics: "Almost 65 percent of U.S. employed adults cite work as a primary source of stress."

This is a time in our history when we have a documented significant increase in hate crimes — prejudice-motivated crimes typically involving violence.

According to the Southern Poverty Law Center in Alabama, "The FBI said law enforcement agencies nationally reported a five-year high in hate crimes, with 6,121 in 2016. That's up over 2015, which saw 5,818 such crimes reported, a near 5% increase." (The full FBI hate crimes statistical report can be found in the resources section at the end of this book.)

There is so much fear on both sides. The folks who are perpetrating the crimes are acting out of fear, and those who are the potential victims are walking around in fear, wondering if they will be the next target. Whether we are responding directly to criminal and violent events on behalf of the community as a first responder, or whether we are on the front lines working to support individuals and groups of people who are disenfranchised, we are at great risk of absorbing trauma, becoming and staying off-balance, and not being able to continue our important work in the world.

Also from the American Psychological Association "Stress in America" report:

> *The uncertainty and unpredictability tied to the future of our nation is affecting the health and well-being of many Americans in a way that feels unique to this period in recent history....*
>
> *More than half of Americans (59 percent) said they consider this the lowest point in U.S. history that they can remember — a figure spanning every generation, including those who lived through World War II and Vietnam, the Cuban Missile Crisis and the Sept. 11 terrorist attacks.*

We cannot underestimate this report and how significant the results are. It matters little whether we are in more danger than ever or whether we are statistically at the lowest point in U.S. history, or how we even define that. What matters most is our perception that this is our reality. Are you feeling this also?

An Ethical and Spiritual Path
If you are reading this book, I know you are committed to an ethical work practice and a balanced and whole life. I know that you are stressed and overwhelmed trying to do it all. I know that you know that being busy and trying to be superhuman is detracting from your wellness and is taking away from your ability to be effective and from your ability to be happy and feel whole. I know this because, when talking with colleagues and other helping professionals as they shared their own stories of stress,

fatigue, fear, and potential burnout, these stories often tied in with their belief in the path they have chosen and their drive to do their work ethically.

I know that our human journey is about being in touch with our spirit, which includes finding and using our unique strengths, gifts, talents, and contributions, and we cannot bring those to fruition if we are not practicing Self-Care. Simultaneously, we all have lessons to learn while on Earth, and we cannot learn those effectively if we are not practicing Self-Care, if we are not balanced and well enough to see the lessons, never mind learn from them. Part of our human journey is to find our unique strengths, gifts, and lessons.

Cathy shared her thoughts on Self-Care as someone who represents several sides of the professional and personal spectrum of caring for others. She is both a clinical mental health counselor and mother to a child (now young man) with significant additional needs. Her story highlights the lack of intention and follow-through with an educational or professional mandate for Self-Care.

> *Self-Care was a familiar word during my graduate work focused on clinical mental health training, then in my work as a clinician, and over the past several years as the parent of a child with special needs. It was never clearly defined; however, we discussed how important self-care was in classes and at professional development meetings, but truly not many people in my circle of support practiced self-care. In fact, I do not remember a time where self-care was encouraged or supported during graduate school, work, or as a parent. It seems to me it is becoming one of those buzzwords — always on my mind and important to encourage others to do, but nothing I had time to practice!*

Cathy now shows how out of control one's life and health can really get when Self-Care is not a priority.

After many episodes of anxiety and migraine headaches that were so bad I was convinced I was having a brain aneurism, I was rushed to the hospital for chest pain and a severe panic attack that took control of me quickly, and the results of thousands of dollars of tests was that I was stressed!

I remember reflecting as I lay in the hospital bed, thinking of what went wrong and wondering what I could do to not repeat this episode again. I knew I had to get better at self-care in order to be the best I could be. Practicing self-care seems to be an ongoing journey, and it feels like it's getting harder in our world today.

By not carrying out any personal Self-Care, Cathy was unable to be of service as a parent and as a mental health professional during her time of extreme stress.

Conclusion

Time magazine's June 6, 1983 cover story called stress, "The Epidemic of the Eighties" and referred to it as America's leading health problem. We are in a considerably worse situation now in 2018. The American Institute of Stress indicates that increased crime, violence, and other threats to personal safety; peer pressure leading to substance abuse; and unhealthy lifestyle habits have all escalated in the intervening decades. Although we live in modern times, our bodies are still responding with the ancient fight-or-flight responses, which are

> *now not only not useful, but potentially damaging and deadly. Repeatedly invoked, it is not hard to see how they can contribute to hypertension, strokes, heart attacks, diabetes, ulcers, neck or low back pain and other "Diseases of Civilization."* (Paul J. Rosch, The American Institute of Stress website)

Helping professionals are the first to respond to incidences of violence, threats, and unhealthy responsive behaviors. It is affecting our work and our personal lives equally. This path is not sustainable. This book is a response to this and a call to action for not only intentional Self-Care but sustainable and sustained Self-Care and Revolutionary Self-Care. This can only happen through awareness, education and professional development, and an active and purposeful change to our work culture.

Two

THE PILLARS

How we care for ourselves gives our brain messages that shape our self-worth, so we must care for ourselves in every way, every day.
Sam Owen, relationship coach

Self-Care as an Act of Justice
Self-Care Revolution is a movement. The *Self-Care Revolution* is about Self-Care as an act of justice in response to our busyness and our fear and our dwindling motivation and lessening love for our work, and for our disappearing balance of work and life. We all need to be well to do good work, to raise our families, to learn our important life lessons, to support and love each other, and to bring to the world our unique gifts, talents, and contributions. There is not a moment more to wait. I believe that as helping professionals, we must value wellness enough that we build our life and professional practice around Self-Care. We must actively move in the direction of wellness, and we must support one another on this path. These are all Revolutionary acts! A Revolution doesn't mean we have to fight. This Revolution is about mindfulness, compassion, intention, and love.

Here are two great definitions of "revolution" in the *Merriam-Webster* online dictionary that we can use to guide our understanding: "a sudden, radical, or complete change" and "a fundamental change in the way of thinking about or visualizing something: a change of paradigm."

Why a Revolution? A Revolution with a capital "R" requires everyone's participation and a marked change of perspective and action. I believe that is exactly what we need when it comes to Self-Care.

Let us stop participating in a system that takes away our energy, our passion, and our compassion. Let us say NO to a world that feeds our fear and our stress. Instead, let us say YES to making a plan to move decidedly and mindfully in the direction of hope, resilience, stability, wellness, and love for ourselves and for others.

Come with me on the Self-Care Revolution journey and find your capacity for sustained resilience and leadership in the Self-Care movement. If you are a social worker, teacher, mental health or other health care provider, clergy, first responder, coach, leader, or anyone feeling stressed and overwhelmed, here are the 5 Pillars I will take you through in this book:

Pillar 1 – Define Self-Care
Pillar 2 – Write a Values Statement
Pillar 3 – Make a Self-Care Plan
Pillar 4 – Recognize Impairment and Focus on Prevention
Pillar 5 – Support Others in Their Self-Care Plans

I believe that we are responsible for ourselves. I believe that we all have our own rhythms, and that knowing and being in our rhythm brings balance, self-confidence, freedom, trust, clarity, and wellness. We can practice Self-Care from our own rhythm. There is not one formula. I also believe that we are accountable to others. We are in community and in relation with everyone on the planet, so someone else's wellness or disease directly affects our own wellness and vice versa. I don't think we can truly be well if we are not supporting wellness for everyone.

One of the best ways you can fight discrimination is by taking good care of yourself. Your survival is not just important; it's an act of revolution.
DaShanne Stokes, author, speaker, civil rights activist

Dylan, a firefighter still early in his career, is seeing a response to the gradual realization and understanding of the critical importance of Self-Care in his firehouse near Boston, Massachusetts. The Firefighter Functional Fitness Guide names four Pillars. They are 1) physical fitness, 2) recovery and rest, 3) hydration, and 4) nutrition and lifestyle. Dylan and his colleagues are taking this very seriously, embedding these practices into their life and work.

> *As a firefighter, without Self-Care, I wouldn't be able to fulfill my obligation to my community. If I can't fulfill that obligation, then in return I wouldn't feel good when I am not working, and vice versa. Proactive care is the best solution to the stress. If firefighters take care of themselves daily, then there will always be less of a chance of injury, mental or physical.*

Dylan makes some strong points about the effectiveness of "proactive care." This is based on the knowledge of the potential ramifications that come with the job of firefighter. This is also based on his value of needing to be at his best in order to be of service.

Conclusion

Self-Care is not just some nice, warm, and cozy concept where we drink tea, attend an occasional yoga class, or check "get together with a friend" off our list of Self-Care to-dos. Self-Care, if revolutionized, means making a fundamental change in our way of relating to ourselves and to one another. It means making a fundamental change in how we see ourselves, each other, and our greater communities and cultures. It means making a fundamental change in our health care system and in our legislation and regulations. If we are determined and committed to being well, to loving ourselves and to loving one another, we can change the course of action. This is a Revolution!

I believe that through intentional and sustained Self-Care we are better able to find and give our unique talents, gifts, and contributions to the world while simultaneously learning our life's lessons. I also believe this is a cyclical process. As we give our best selves, we are mindful to learn our lessons, and in this space we are inherently practicing sustained Self-Care.

Three

Pillar 1: Define Self-Care

There's only one corner of the universe you can be certain of improving, and that's your own self.
Aldous Huxley, writer, philosopher, humanist, pacifist

The idea that we have control only over ourselves is fundamental. I believe that we each have a responsibility to be our best self while on the planet. I am so committed to this idea. It's not easy to be committed to this, because all of my decisions center around this belief.

"Am I being my best? Am I doing my best? Am I making my greatest contribution?"

These are the questions I ask myself every day. I also believe that I cannot be and do my best unless I am living within the framework of Self-Care. We can't improve on our Self-Care if we don't really know what the term means to us. Before getting too deep into this Pillar, I'd like you to do some brainstorming. For each Pillar you will be asked to complete an initial assessment: What do you know now? What do you think now? At the end of each Pillar, you will be asked to complete a post-assessment: What do you know now? What do you think now? The difference between the initial assessment and the post-assessment will allow you to easily see your learning, growth, and insight just from reading the Pillar information. You can complete these assessments in the workbook found later in this manuscript.

Pillar 1: Define Self-Care — Initial Assessment
Take a few minutes to jot down in your workbook what Self-Care is and means to you. Avoid the urge to look up any definitions. Keep in mind that Self-Care is personal and cultural and has the capacity to move and change with us over time, and this is just your initial assessment of what you know and think in this moment. Your definition is not set in stone,

and when you start to put things in writing you may see things that might be quite different than what you imagined in your head. Perhaps at one point you thought Self-Care was one thing, but now you think it may be something different. Let your ideas flow without judgment.

Try these prompts if you don't know where to start.

Think about your five senses. What does Self-Care feel like, look like, smell like, taste like, sound like to you? What are the key themes, ideas, and words that come up for you when you hear the term "Self-Care"? Fill in the blank: "When I do _____, I feel good." Think broadly!

1) What does Self-Care mean to you?
2) How do you define Self-Care now?

Self-Care Is Cultural and Personal

What one person or culture considers to be Self-Care is not necessarily what another considers to be so. Also, when Self-Care is defined in relation to social justice, it can have an even more revolutionary importance. Self-Care can be both preventative as well as reactional. We may have different definitions of Self-Care for different categories, like environmental Self-Care or psychological Self-Care. Some cultures are much more tied to their natural environments and may more closely identify with environmental Self-Care. Some individuals may closely align themselves with spiritual practices like meditation or prayer, and those may factor more strongly in their Self-Care definition, while others favor cardio exercise and being physically active. If we live in a culture that values being vegetarian, our food choices will likely factor into our definition of Self-Care. This is highly personal and cultural, and there is no right or wrong definition of Self-Care.

My Self-Care and Self-Management

How do I define Self-Care? My Self-Care does include things like candles and baths and massages and pedicures, the more typical types of Self-Care that help people, including myself, to feel pampered and taken care of and, at least temporarily, relaxed! I have candles all over my house. I have one on my desk, and its presence adds a level of aesthetic value to my work space that makes a tangible difference. I get a monthly massage and they are always scheduled a month ahead of time. Do I always get to keep that appointment? Often as the date gets closer, I have to reschedule, but I am usually able to schedule it within a day or two.

As a person who has been managing chronic pain since young childhood, everything I do in the name of Self-Care feels like it is for body, mind, and spirit. I can barely separate one from the other, as they are so intertwined; they affect one another intimately. If I am relaxed in my mind, my body is more relaxed. If my body is more relaxed, I will have less pain, and managing my pain is one of my self-management pieces. Another self-management piece to my Self-Care is my work as a helping professional. We all have that self-management piece in common. Our work is a pre-existing condition that we have to take into consideration when we define and practice Self-Care.

My Self-Care also includes paying attention to my finances, my work-life fit, my employment and paid-work endeavors, the time I spend on self-growth, and in general all the time I devote to my life choices. Every decision I make is a Self-Care decision. It requires me to constantly check in. "Does this serve me? Is this my path? Does it feel good? Is there something missing, or not quite right? Is this something I can or need to do on my own or do I need help and support?"

My biggest struggle with Self-Care is between time and money. By nature I am someone who likes to get things done. I want to be efficient and effective with my time and efforts. I have high expectations for myself and always want to be at my best, doing my best. I also always seem to be anxious about money, no matter if I have enough or not. This puts a stress on my decisions of how to spend my time. For me, Self-Care is an everyday part of life that includes what I put on my body, what I put in my body, how I exercise and move, how I spend my time, who I spend my time with, and how my decisions and efforts are serving me and my path.

As I have mentioned, I strongly believe that we are all here with unique gifts, talents, and contributions and that we all have lessons to learn. For me, the ultimate Self-Care is determining these gifts, talents, contributions, and lessons, and doing everything in their name, for their sake. Self-Care is the ultimate "Why am I here?" I don't want to miss my opportunities to give or to receive. My mindfulness of this is how I ultimately define Self-Care.

I have come by this definition through a long and sometimes painful journey, but through the pain I have found my abilities to be mindful and to understand the complexities of Self-Care, as well as the breadth and depth of what Self-Care can be. Most importantly, I have come to accept and honor that it is indeed a journey, even one that is messy and bumpy. I think of it as a balance in the long run.

I may not be balanced every day, or even every week, but I ask myself, "How am I doing this month? This year? Am I living my values? Am I honoring my unique gifts, talents, and contributions? Am I learning my lessons?"

If I've already learned a lesson, the moment or experience will feel easy and I will feel good. In parenting my son, I have found many moments of gratitude for my learning, as I am able to take a deep breath instead of losing my patience or spending the extra time in the morning getting ready, even if it means having to shift how the rest of the day goes. If I haven't yet learned a lesson, the moment or experience will feel hard. The ease or difficulty of this feeling and this moment are not because I am out of balance; they are because I haven't learned this lesson yet. In my work as a recovering perfectionist, learning that often "good enough" is really good enough is a hard lesson for me. I have made substantial strides, but this lesson can still bite me. I can get caught up in a moment when I have trouble letting something go, either for myself or an expectation of someone else. The Self-Care comes in when I can be mindful and recognize this moment as an opportunity. "Why does this feel hard? What am I supposed to be paying attention to?" Being mindful in these moments is a way to "sit with the hard" and to ensure that I learn my lessons so I have fewer hard moments as the years move on. When it's obvious that the same lesson continues to repeat itself, this is one of my greatest opportunities for self-compassion. In the challenge of this is incredible potential to learn how to love.

I work hard to be the best version of myself in the most balanced way, and being my best is part of my Self-Care. I know I cannot please everyone. I know I cannot always please myself. Being my best means being mindful of my lessons when they arise and having self-compassion and self-love to help guide me to learn those lessons. Being my best means taking the best care of myself possible and also supporting others to be their best. I know in my heart that this is the way forward.

Matthew, an urgent-care nurse practitioner in his mid-career, is a practicing Muslim. There are Pillars to his Muslim faith that help guide his Self-Care, although he hadn't thought about these Muslim Pillars in relation to Self-Care before our conversation. He said this about his definition of Self-Care as he made the connections in his head and heart while we chatted:

> *One aspect of Self-Care to me is knowing that the most certain thing in life, which is death, could occur at any time in a person's life regardless of age. Once I die, all the things that I have been working hard my whole life to achieve do not go to the grave with me. Knowing death could occur at any time without warning teaches me to be nice to strangers, friends, and family alike, and this is fundamentally part of my Self-Care.*

His Muslim faith gives him Pillars of reference to base his life decisions on. These Pillars are the foundation of his definition of Self-Care, including his concept of death and how that faith manifests in his daily actions with those around him.

I love how my actions of love and service to others and his actions of being nice to strangers, friends, and family are in parallel, even though they come from different values. Both factor into our individual definitions of Self-Care.

Other Formal Definitions of Self-Care

I want you to consider Self-Care in the broadest of ways. There have been a series of definitions of Self-Care over the years put out by health-focused and Self-Care-focused organizations. Here are a couple to review as you further refine how you might define Self-Care for yourself. This one aligns with part of my definition and approach to Self-Care that includes self-management.

> *The focus of the International Self-Care Foundation is on self-care in the preservation of wellness in healthy people, to help prevent the epidemic of lifestyle diseases. This is where the greatest need lies currently. However, it is important to emphasize that self-care is also essential for people with an existing disease condition, and this is also sometimes referred to as "self-management" of the condition. Self-care is also usually the first treatment response to everyday health conditions and common ailments. Self-care is therefore the fundamental level of health care in all societies and should be seen as a major public health resource. Yet self-care is often unrecognized and underappreciated.* (International Self-Care Foundation website)

As someone with chronic pain, I have spent all my life managing my health and wellness, otherwise known as "self-management." I believe everyone has some self-management component to their Self-Care. For those of us in the helping professions, our work itself is one self-management component to our Self-Care.

Because I had a lot of physical symptoms for a long time with no diagnosis, I learned early on the importance of Self-Care in the context of "first treatment response," as mentioned. It also became increasingly challenging emotionally and psychologically. I had to be my own doctor, my own massage therapist, my own therapist, and my own advocate.

I have learned to find doctors and medical professionals who are willing and able to be on my team. I spend the necessary time setting up appointments with different doctors and healing providers to find the one who understands that I am a crusader for my Self-Care but that I am also looking for help and support. I know I can't do it on my own and I don't want to. I had a primary care practitioner for a number of years who was my partner in health and wellness. I asked her if she would partner with me in my commitment to my Self-Care. I brought her the information and asked my questions and we brainstormed together, decided on tests to do or not do, discussed potential treatment options, and in general established how best to move forward. I have had this kind of relationship with many different health practitioners, including a craniosacral therapist, a psychologist, more than one massage therapist, an acupuncturist, and a naturopath. I consider my practitioners to be part of my team.

This is often a challenge. It is time-consuming and often frustrating. I often don't get the information I am looking or hoping for. Sometimes I get stuck in a loop of searching for answers. This happens when I am having a flare-up of pain. I have gained so much knowledge and expertise on how to take care of myself, I wind up feeling annoyed with myself for getting stuck in the loop of searching. In this loop I find my own wisdom gained and I find my life's lessons.

One lesson I continue to learn is self-compassion and self-love. It's okay to search for answers. It's okay to ask for help. It's okay that sometimes I search outside myself when I already know the answers. My Self-Care path has not only been transformational for myself, it has forged my path as a social worker, educator, healing professional, metaphysical minister, musician, and now author.

The following World Health Organization (WHO) definition is focused on Self-Care as it relates to physical health and the prevention and limiting of illness and disease. This may speak to some more than others as you consider your own definition. For me, this piece of the Self-Care equation is incredibly important, as it also supports my self-management activities to partner with my health providers. Do you see elements of your own definition emerging out of WHO's definition?

> *Self Care in health refers to the activities individuals, families and communities undertake with the intention of*

enhancing health, preventing disease, limiting illness, and restoring health. These activities are derived from knowledge and skills from the pool of both professional and lay experience. They are undertaken by lay people on their own behalf, either separately or in participative collaboration with professionals. (World Health Organization, "Health Education in Self-Care: Possibilities and Limitations")

Self-Care as Social Justice

I believe that at our most basic level we are spiritual beings living in human bodies. I believe we all have the need to take care of ourselves (body, mind, soul) and the responsibility of helping others on their Self-Care path. We are connected and in this together. We can only be well if all are supported to be well. When one person claims his or her power by committing to Self-Care, everyone benefits.

Self-Care is non-hierarchical, and in some ways this is an equalizer, because it applies to everyone. Yet in other ways, there are some on this planet who need more because of where they are born or the color of their skin, poverty, homeless status, illness, lack of insurance or access to education or health care, and others. One way we can advocate and help others find empowerment is through the act of Self-Care and our service to others for their Self-Care. It is something everyone can do and it is something everyone can feel empowered to be in control of, in some way. It is also something that everyone can feel supported to do.

Self-Care goes way beyond lighting candles, taking baths, and getting a massage.

If our culture supports us to be unwell and to stay unwell, and we respond by fiercely taking back control of our wellness with a sustainable commitment to Self-Care that includes supporting others' Self-Care, we are acting in service of ourselves, our families, and our communities. It would mean a fundamental change in our way of relating to ourselves and to one another.

Women report higher rates of stress than men, and people of color report higher rates of stress than white people. Why? Women and people of color are marginalized and have to work harder to overcome more barriers. They have to explain and defend their existence and their importance, and this takes away critical energy that they cannot then use on their own Self-Care. For them to practice Self-Care then becomes an act of justice, to say, "I am important. I am just as important as you are. It is not my responsibility to explain to you my history, the injustices, my worth. It is up to me to stay well."

> *Caring for myself is not self-indulgence, it is self-preservation, and that is an act of political warfare.*
> Audre Lorde, social justice advocate

The definitions and approach of the Self Care Forum in the UK support Self-Care as social justice; its mandate also supports my Self-Care Revolution. The Forum's definition includes actions on behalf of and with others, and sees self-empowerment and collective process as ways toward systemic change. I see Self-Care as an act of justice that includes individual spirituality, includes supporting others in their Self-Care, and ultimately creates transformational societies.

> *The actions that individuals take for themselves, on behalf of and with others in order to develop, protect, maintain and improve their health, wellbeing or wellness.... A radical act of justice to preserve the soul, spirit, and well-being of an individual to self-empower others and contribute to transformative societal change.* (Self Care Forum website)

These concepts and approaches to Self-Care — to be focused on developing, protecting, maintaining, and improving wellness; to preserve the spirit of the individual; to facilitate and support people's empowerment; and to contribute to transformative societal change — are all critical to the Self-Care Revolution.

Cathy, the counselor and parent of a child with significant special needs whom we met in chapter one, came to a critical point in her life as it relates to Self-Care.

> *My self-care was crucial to my survival in the world as a human being and I could no longer keep moving at a pace too fast for myself. I needed a place and time to connect with myself. I learned to weave in self-care each day by carving out a space in my life where no one was putting any demands on me, not even myself — that is my personal definition of self-care.*

Ashley, the child protective investigator from chapter one, defines Self-Care this way:

> *Self-care, for me, can be the result of self-discipline. As an example, reading a book instead of sitting in front of the TV is more restful. Yet I had been in a mindless routine of sitting in front of the TV every night. It's easier to just sit in front of the TV and pick up the remote, easier because it had become a habit. Perhaps creating another habit around the things I enjoy, like reading or sewing, would become just as easy. I have told myself I don't have time for the things I enjoy doing, but I think for me it really boils down to discipline.*

Do you see yourself in any of these stories and examples of Self-Care definitions? What fits for you? How is your personal definition shaping up in your head? What professional and personal stories of your own can you pull from to summarize an operational Self-Care definition for yourself?

Pillar 1: Define Self-Care — Post-Assessment
You will need to go to your workbook for this exercise.

Looking back through this chapter and looking at your workbook and your initial assessment of defining Self-Care, would you make any changes to how you define Self-Care based on your reading or any new understandings? Take a look at the answers to your assessment questions, review the organizational and personal definitions presented, and refine your own definition here. This will be your working definition. You can change it at any time. It is never set in stone.

Conclusion
Be flexible and go easy on yourself. The definition you come up with for yourself in this chapter does not have to be the definition you maintain throughout your life. As you learn, grow, perhaps change jobs or even careers, and continue to practice Self-Care through all of it, you may find you need to adjust your definition. Keep it handy and consider assessing your definition once a year, or at a minimum when you are going through, about to face, or have just made a major life change.

These are critical times to assess our lives and ourselves at all levels, with Self-Care being one of the most important components of our lives that needs attention. I recommend assessing your Self-Care definition before making a major life decision. How does this new life change affect your Self-Care? Can your definition help you make a better decision, the best decision?

Four

Pillar 2: Write a Values Statement

Values are like fingerprints. Nobody's are the same, but you leave 'em all over everything you do.
Elvis Presley, singer, film star

What Is Your "Why"?
Have you defined the "why" of your life and work? We are often asked, "What do you do?" Our responses most often refer to what we do for regular paid employment. Rarely will someone respond to this by talking about their hobbies or passions if they lie outside what they do for paid employment. Even more rarely does the conversation move toward the more important question of "Why?"

A mission statement states what you do and who and what you do this for. The mission is the overall purpose. A vision statement describes the future you are working toward, ideally your final desired end state. A Values Statement answers why you do what you do and for whom. Values are a compass to guide your actions and decisions. Why do you do what you do? Why do you make the decisions you make?

We will always feel out of balance and out of rhythm if what we do is different from what we believe in. This speaks loudly to me of Self-Care as a value. If I believe Self-Care is of utmost importance, I will think about it. I will grow in my self-compassion and self-love and my mindfulness of caring for myself. I will practice Self-Care. I will learn better how to value my Self-Care and all that it entails and all that it has to offer. Valuing Self-Care and therefore practicing Self-Care will bring me satisfaction and fulfillment.

The *Oxford English Dictionary* defines "values" this way: "the regard that something is held to deserve; the importance, worth, or usefulness of something; a person's principles or standards of behavior; one's judgment of what is important in life."

One's behaviors are the outward expressions of what one values. Take a minute to assess where you stand in your personal life and in your current work life. Have you ever considered what your core values are? What guides your life and your decisions, including your work? If this is something you have never done, I strongly encourage you to consider this in this moment. In the space you are in reading this book and considering Self-Care at a different level, take a minute to consider the why of your life.

Remember, these are just assessment exercises to get you thinking and to give you an idea of where you stand. No one else ever has to see your work here.

You may ask yourself, "Why should I consider crafting a personal Values Statement?" My answer is, to find your why. It can be an incredibly powerful tool for how you live your life, what decisions you make, and how you feel about yourself. Therefore, it will predict how well you practice Self-Care. Your values are your why.

Pillar 2: Write a Values Statement — Initial Assessment

You will need your workbook for this exercise.

Start by writing a list of what you value. Don't censor yourself. This is a brainstorm. You probably won't put anything on the list that you don't inherently value, but a lengthy list doesn't mean you have to include all of them in a statement.

Here are some examples of values: ethics, excellence, diversity, inclusivity, honesty, innovation, collaboration, excitement, freedom, sustainability, fun, cleanliness, integrity, simplicity, loyalty, service, compassion, hope, and of course Self-Care, wellness, balance, and health. Other examples of things we value are family, friends, home ownership, and independence.

You might want to choose your top three or four values and write one statement using all of them. You might alternatively choose to write one statement for each. It's entirely up to you. Part of a sustainable Self-

Care Plan is to create a Values Statement for yourself and include Self-Care in it in some capacity, or create an entire Values Statement just for Self-Care. You don't necessarily need to use the word "Self-Care." You might use "wellness" or "balance" or "health" or something along those lines that you value, where you would have to practice Self-Care in order to live that value.

How do you get from your list of Values to a Values Statement? Remember that your behaviors and actions are guided by your values. What do you believe in? What do you hold to be true? A Values Statement reflects what is most important to you.

It can be helpful to consider your strengths and what you are good at, as often this is closely aligned with your values. Think about your successes and times in your life when you feel you are in rhythm with your best self. What values are reflected in those successes? What behaviors do you value in others? What ways of being in relationship with others do you value? What do you value about your favorite company or restaurant? When you shop or eat out at your favorite spots, what makes them feel good? How are you treated? Think about your jobs and about what made your best job the best. Was it because you were living and working from your values? Were your values in alignment with your employer's?

Look for evidence of your values in your behaviors and life choices and experiences.

Here are some examples of Values Statements:

"We operate by the following guiding principles: Honesty, Integrity, Customer Service, Quality, Diversity and Innovation."
"We work from a place of honesty, integrity, and openness in all we do."
"We value equitable collaboration."
"We value the uniqueness of people, perspectives, and abilities."
"We value and encourage personal development."
"We value being of service in a caring manner."
"We value inspiration and a vision for all the good that is possible."
"We are professional, ethical, innovative, and available."
"We value environmental responsibility."

Self-Care Equation

> *Imagine a world where we wake up inspired to go to work. Why do you get up in the morning? Why does your organization exist? Your Why is the purpose, cause or belief that inspires you to do what you do. When you think, act and communicate starting with "Why," you can inspire others.* (Simon Sinek, Ted Talk)

This is Simon Sinek's equation: Values x Behavior = Culture

I will take this one step further. This is my Self-Care Equation:

Values x Behavior = Self-Care

When you think, act, and communicate starting with your values, you are practicing one of the best forms of Self-Care. It also means that if you put Self-Care in your Values Statement in some way, it will help you bring your unique talents, gifts, and contributions to the world as your best self.

I believe that through intentional and sustained Self-Care we are better able to find and give our unique talents, gifts, and contributions to the world while simultaneously learning our life's lessons. I also believe this is a cyclical process. As we give our best selves, we are mindful to learn our lessons, and in this space we are inherently practicing sustained Self-Care. This is what this equation, **Values x Behavior = Self-Care** means.

If you define your values and live out your life based on those values, you are practicing the most comprehensive form of Self-Care, dare I say radical and revolutionary Self-Care. Every decision you make every day can be in the name of Self-Care. Ask yourself, "Does it match my values? Is it really what I want or need to do? Does it support my mission and vision? Will it make me feel good, or will it put me in a state of dis-ease?"

When I make a decision that matches my values, it is in my best interest. I feel good about the decision and I feel even better about the result of the decision. I feel in alignment with myself and the Universe. I feel free and inspired and energized. I feel empowered to continue to make those decisions that best serve my values, because I want to feel like that all the time!

Do you know the feeling? Have you had this feeling?

It can be something simple, such as showing up to a concert that was on your schedule to attend but you didn't really feel like you had the energy to make it happen. These moments can be tricky to navigate. Is it Self-Care to attend the concert or Self-Care to rest and stay home? I think it depends, and the answer will be different each time. In these moments we can be quietly and mindfully with ourselves to determine the best outcome. What I do is imagine myself at the concert and imagine myself staying home. What would each feel like? Look like? When I imagine myself at the concert (or gym or party or work or insert whatever makes sense to you here), I can feel in my body and mind whether the best thing for me at that moment is rallying to attend or hunkering down at home.

On the other hand, we can make decisions that make us feel anxious and take up an enormous amount of mental energy, trying to figure out what we are doing and why we found ourselves in this position. In these moments we are not feeling free or in alignment, but very much the opposite. We are questioning our work, our lives, our choices, sometimes our very existence, and in these moments we might question our values.

Going back to my basic belief system that we all have lessons we need to learn while we are here on Earth, I believe these are the key moments for learning. I think sometimes we make a decision that goes against our values, and we might have had the capacity to make a different choice. I think, though, that most of the time we generally make the only decision we can at the time and then it is up to us to learn from that. This is also Self-Care. It is in the awareness and the mindfulness of our lessons in these moments that we are practicing Self-Care.

Here is Matthew again, our mid-career urgent-care nurse practitioner who is a devout practicing Muslim:

> *Self-Care for me cannot be described without incorporating many aspects of my Islamic beliefs. My beliefs as a Muslim encompass all aspects of my daily activities. I will begin with the morning routine, which includes my early*

> *morning prayer.... [T]he morning call to prayer ... is how my day starts, and this sequence is repeated five times a day. So regardless of how bad of a day I am having, at some point I have to stop what I am doing and pray, which is a kind of reset or a check on whatever is going on. My prayers reset my attitude if I am feeling overwhelmed.*

His religion guides his values, which guide his Self-Care and care of others as a medical practitioner. He begins each daily activity with a phrase,

> Bismillah al-rahman al-rahim, [which means] *"in the Name of Allah Most Gracious Most Merciful." I do it with eating, talking with patients, etc. This makes me God-conscious and makes me aware that although my day might be bad, there is the distinct possibility that my day is not as bad as the person next to me; hence, be grateful for what I have.*

Living his Muslim values is the basis for his definition and practicing of Self-Care. This also demonstrates a mindful approach to living and moving through the world. The mindfulness is part of his Self-Care. This level of mindfulness speaks to his compassion for himself, for his clients, and for his community. It also speaks of love. His prayers and his focus on his faith give him compassion and love for himself and others. This feeds his Self-Care and makes him a loving and able medical professional. Some may question his practice of praying five times a day and wonder how he can take the time to keep up with that, but Matthew is able to move through his days staying grounded because this practice is deeply embedded into his life. These moments of prayer ground him for what comes next in his job and in his life.

How well do you know and understand your employer's values? What if your values don't match up with your employer's values? How does this factor into your Self-Care? How long do you stay with an employer whose values don't align with yours? How is this misalignment manifesting in your life and work? How do you choose which jobs to even apply for in the first place?

Having a Values Statement is a great way to be able to discern what employers and jobs would be a good match for you. It's also a great way to begin preparing for a successful interview. Prepare to talk about yourself and your strengths by talking about your values and your why. What is behind all that you have done and accomplished? Your values. Is this also true of your employer?

One of my mentors, Pam, is a clergyperson in higher education. She is new in my life, but I have come to value and rely on her insights.

> *In order to have Self-Care for yourself, you have to have a sense of self-respect, and in order to have self-respect, you have to be at peace with who you are. Otherwise, you feel shame or guilt or pain about yourself and you aren't going to treat yourself very well. It has a lot to do with living in sync with the person you imagine yourself to be at its best, in sync with the values you hold. When we live out of that framework, we cause ourselves pain and guilt and shame.*

She took values even one step further as she talked about action and the distinction between values and virtues.

> *I have a very clear distinction, though, between what do I value and what do I practice. This is the distinction between values and virtues. Virtues are something that are always practiced. Virtues we build up over time. Courage is a virtue (this is Maya Angelou's insight). We are not born with courage, but it is something we can learn through taking risks. We practice it. If I value something, in what way do I embody it? I value justice, but in what ways am I practicing and living into that value? I want to claim it. I want to work on it, struggle with it. This is all part of Self-Care for me.*

This is powerful for me because it took Values to another level. I had not thought of virtues or the difference between values and virtues. I have spent some time considering this for myself and how I might differentiate between my values and virtues. I think often we talk about values when we might mean virtues, but there is also some difference as it relates to cultural norms versus personal traits. We value things in terms of cultural norms, such as being on time or dressing up for special occasions. We tend to practice virtues as personal characteristics, such as being honest or being kind. On another note, I value my family, so how do I behave in a way that embodies that value?

As I delve more into this, it seems there is a lot of overlap between what you might value and what you practice, as in a virtue. I value honesty and therefore I practice honesty. I value wellness, so I practice Self-Care. In light of this new understanding, I invite you to consider this. You may have things you value, like being on time, that are partly cultural but that you ascribe less importance to than a value that is more of a personal characteristic, like being brave.

I suggest you focus, when writing your Values Statement, on the Values that you practice as an outward expression of who you are and what you believe in. I would focus on your Values Statement under the umbrella of "My Why." Ask yourself, "Why do I do what I do?" Because you value wellness? Because you value community and being in relation with others? Because you value diversity and equality?

Pillar 2: Write a Values Statement — Post-Assessment
You will need your workbook for this exercise.

Now that you have brainstormed your list of Values, written a first draft of one or several Values Statements, and read the whole Pillar 2 chapter, you are ready to edit and polish your final Values Statement(s). Take a look at your first version. Does anything need to be completely changed, or does it just need a small tweak? Maybe you will leave it as is. If so, just rewrite it. You can always come back to this and change it as needed. This is yours.

Conclusion

After reading this chapter, considering the definitions and examples provided, and looking back at your workbook to your initial assessment, you have now also taken some time to edit or rewrite your initial draft Values Statement(s). As always, remember to give yourself a lot of leeway. No one can define your Values but you. This means you get to change them if they need changing. Don't get too bogged down. This Pillar exercise itself, regardless of the result, will have been incredibly valuable.

We will tackle goals and strategies to reaching those goals in "Pillar 3: Make a Self-Care Plan."

Five

Pillar 3: Make a Self-Care Plan

By Failing to Prepare, You are Preparing to Fail.
Benjamin Franklin, author, political theorist,
scientist, inventor, humorist, civic activist

So now, with a working definition of Self-Care and a working Values Statement for your life and your work, you are ready to make a Self-Care Plan. For this Pillar, you will start with an assessment, then you will consider strengths, barriers, and priorities, and look at three stories from professionals to help understand Self-Care Plans within a context. Finally, you will sketch out a Self-Care Plan for yourself!

Don't get too caught up in your definitions at this point. If you went through the assessments and exercises for Pillars 1 and 2, you have something to work from. This can always be changed as you delve deeper into your Self-Care and live a life based on your values. There is no right or wrong, and no final definition. This is a living, breathing process that is part of your life's work, and it can change as you grow and change. It is meant to be your guide. It is not meant to be a straitjacket!

During the writing of this book I am getting much clearer about my own specifics, as I have to think about them differently in order to write them down comprehensively and systematically. Every time you write something down, you will gain clarity. Every time you are mindful and intentional about your Self-Care assessment, your plan will also become clearer. I would expect that, over time, your plan will change. You will need different things at different times.

Take the self-care assessment through my website, www.ellenrondina.com/self-care before going to your workbook to complete the Pillar 3 assessment. If you haven't already done this, it will give you a starting point, help you to identify your gaps in knowledge of your practice of

Self-Care, and give you some more ideas about what you can put into your plan for it to be intentional and sustainable!

Once you complete the assessment and submit, you will receive by email a guide to what your results mean and some suggestions for how to view your results.

Pillar 3: Make a Self-Care Plan — Initial Assessment
You will need your workbook for this.

What are you currently doing for Self-Care? Do you have any kind of specific or regular plan? Do you have a goal for your Self-Care? Even if you don't have a written plan or goal, or have never thought of it before, take a minute to jot down everything you can think of that you do that you would consider Self-Care in each of the labeled categories: physical, spiritual, psychological, emotional, relational, professional, and environmental, as well as maintenance Self-Care and emergency Self-Care. Remember that Self-Care is comprehensive and covers many areas of our life.

Example Plans
Here is a very specific Self-Care Plan from a mid-career emergency room doctor, Rachel, who had a very intense experience that led her to question her competence and her interest in continuing with her line of work. She titled her plan, "Plan for Resolution of Malaise." This is a resolution plan rather than a prevention plan. Rachel came to this plan after a significant event that followed a period of trauma and burnout with her work.

> *I was feeling a bit ... inept, out of date, rusty, dusty, or just like I was totally not on my game. I was seeing patients and feeling nervous, exhausted, and just not having a great day.*

Her day went from bad to worse and ended with a patient dying. Needless to say, she and her team did their thorough ethical assessment and determined that this patient had in fact been very ill when coming into their emergency room and was not going to survive.

This is the written plan she came up with following this traumatic incident, where she was forced to come to terms with her burnout:
1) *Identify specific concerns and problems and what I consider to be my own areas of weakness.*
2) *Patient satisfaction: What does my supervisor have to say? What are my patients saying? How can I feel confident and well enough to receive critical feedback?*
3) *Make learning and continuing medical education a higher priority: Get recertified.*
4) *Plan for career change (which I discussed with my boss but have since reconsidered).*
5) *Personal wellness (note its place at #5 and that my health insurance covers NONE of the expenses related to this task, which is my top priority in order to prevent dis-ease):*
   * *Psychotherapy (my insurance does not cover this)*
   * *Exercise: yoga, hiking*
   * *Physical health: I saw a chiropractor and massage therapist (my health insurance did not cover either)*

This doc says that the plan is working (so far), but the responsibility and expense is entirely hers. She would love to take a much-needed full retreat, but again that would be another out-of-pocket expense and it would be taking her away from her work and her family, which would ultimately be very difficult to do. Ultimately she would prefer to have a Self-Care prevention plan in order to avoid any repeat situations in her work.

> *It would be such a relief to make prevention of these types of situations a priority to employers and to keep providers providing!*

Organizations' Self-Care Plans

Of course, when we talk about making Self-Care Plans we need to have our individual plans, but the organizations we work for also need to have plans. Just as we want to consider an organization's values when we consider who to work for, we also want to consider if a potential employer has taken their values one step further and has a Self-Care or wellness plan for employees. As you move deeper into establishing Self-Care as a permanent and sustainable foundation in your life and work, you might become more out of rhythm with an employer who is not walking the Self-Care talk.

The Washington Coalition of Sexual Assault Programs is one of those organizations that walks the Self-Care talk. It is a nonprofit organization that brings together agencies engaged in eliminating sexual violence, and it values Self-Care by offering these ideas for how organizations can support Self-Care:

- *Integrate Self-Care activities into your strategic plan.*
- *Create an explicit policy that highlights the organizational value of Self-Care and identifies permissible activities.*
- *Include education about vicarious trauma and Self-Care in the orientation process and ongoing training.*
- *Set up regular opportunities for Self-Care as part of the office routine, such as "check-ins" about well-being during staff meetings, opportunities to debrief after particularly stressful interactions, supervisor-approved time to relax and process difficult concerns, mentorship between staff members, and access to additional supervision time in response to heightened stress.*
- *Don't forget FUN! Including fun activities in meetings and retreats is not frivolous. We need fun to recharge.*
- *Remember to model positive Self-Care. When managers take good care of themselves, the organization benefits. Spa day, anyone?*

These tips really speak to my 5 Pillars. They include making a plan, integrating Self-Care into the values of the organization, providing the time and space to engage in Self-Care activities, and taking a leadership position by a top-down system of modeling Self-Care for all employees to follow suit. Does your employer have a plan for wellness and Self-Care? If not, why not? If so, what does it look like?

What do you want your Self-Care Plan to look like? Here are three areas to think about and strategize around in preparation for writing up a sustainable and effective Self-Care Plan: 1) focus on your strengths, 2) identify any barriers, and 3) take the time to prioritize.

Focus on Your Strengths
You will need your workbook for this section.

Make a list of all your strengths. Here are some prompts to help you:

What do you do well? What are your unique gifts, talents, and contributions in the world? What comes naturally? What do you know how to do? What gives you confidence? What do people compliment you for? Name three of your positive characteristics. Build on these strengths when you create your Self-Care Plan. What do you enjoy? What feeds you? Where, when, and how do you thrive? This is the best place to start.

Next, think about the strengths of your surroundings. What is easily available to you? What is accessible? What is aesthetically pleasing? Where do you go that you enjoy?
Write down as many of your strengths as you can think of in your workbook.

I believe when you are operating from a strengths perspective, you *are* practicing Self-Care. How often are you living your strengths? How often are you functioning and working and moving through the world using these strengths? If you notice that you aren't using your strengths as often as you could, can you make any adjustments? Compare your list of strengths to the results of your Self-Care assessment. If you were practicing from more of a strengths perspective, would you be doing more things "well" in some areas that you marked as doing "okay" or "barely at all"?

Identify Barriers

You will need to consider what your barriers are to practicing Self-Care. What are your barriers to Self-Care and planning for it? What are you struggling with? Why do you really believe you haven't solved the problem of not being attentive to Self-Care? What beliefs about your current situation do you know are getting in the way of moving forward? The biggest mistakes people make when they attempt to change a behavior are these:

    1) not identifying the barriers and, therefore,

    2) not planning on how to get over, past, or around those barriers.

Change involves learning from confronting the obstacles we encounter! And remember, as much as it hurts to be honest about this, change is NOT linear! Change is also not necessarily "failure versus success." Be careful to remember the difference between "This was a failure" and "I am a failure." When it comes to Self-Care, first on our list is to suspend judgment and to be kind — yes, kind to yourself! In other words, you must have compassion and love for yourself.

If you are reading this book, you might be at some kind of fork in the road. The fork is your chance to make decisions, make changes, and experiment with new possibilities. Real change requires a change in belief. The way to bring about sustainable change in belief is through reflection. Consider these concepts of reflection:

    1) Dissatisfaction with the old idea is necessary.

    2) Intelligibility: How will a new strategy work for me?

    3) Plausibility: The new idea has to make sense and be possible.

    4) Fruitfulness: Can I see the advantage of adopting the new concept? How will it enhance or improve my life?

When it comes to Self-Care, are you dissatisfied with your current plan and action? Do you have a notion of how a new Self-Care Plan will work for you? Does creating a different kind of Self-Care Plan make sense to you? Do you believe this will change your life? Do you believe that taking Self-Care to a radically different level, and having and being able to take intentional action on a written plan, will make it a sustainable reality that brings wellness and passion and energy back to your life and to your professional practice?

One mid-career veterinarian, Amy, who owns her own practice in rural Maine, talks about her Self-Care and considers time her "biggest enemy." In general, Amy says, she simply works too many hours. This is her dream career, but she says she is simply doing "too much of it." She is not where she wants to be in her Self-Care, but she has implemented some strategies as part of her current plan.

> *My staff know that I prioritize myself by going for regular massages and taking the time out of my day regularly to do what I enjoy, which is training the dogs.*

She is currently working on expanding her Self-Care Plan, and part of her plan is to hire a personal assistant for a few hours a week and delegate more of the stuff that can be delegated. She would also like to schedule a vacation, but as a practitioner and business owner, this is much more difficult to do. She has not been able to find a relief veterinarian, which is one of her identified barriers to her Self-Care Plan.

> *My fear right now is that if I grow* [my business practice] *to the point where I can afford an associate, I won't be able to find anyone.*

She feels like she is stuck. She doesn't have the support she needs from colleagues in her field and she doesn't know quite how to move forward without the support or without knowing that support will be there when she needs it. In order for her to get around this barrier, she is going to have to do some legwork to identify someone, or multiple people, who might be available and interested in being her associate in her practice. Doing this legwork may in fact highlight some additional barriers, but it also may yield faster results than she expects.

Another barrier for Amy is that veterinary medicine is often not perceived to be a stressful helping profession, which means support and understanding can be lacking.

> *Sources of stress that create poor wellness in veterinarians include giving bad news, managing adverse events, interacting with difficult clients, working in teams, and balancing work and home life. But handling ethical dilemmas is the worst stressor, and research indicates that veterinarians face ethical dilemmas three to five times per week.* (Susan C. Kahler, "Moral stress the top trigger in veterinarians' compassion fatigue")

Here are some other examples of barriers that other professionals have shared as they contemplated their Self-Care:

I am not a morning person and the only time I would have to myself to work out or meditate is in the morning.

I don't have the childcare I need to schedule any more time for myself.

I work for an employer who doesn't value Self-Care, so the expectation is for me to never take time off.

I don't have any extra cash for any kind of Self-Care.

I'm not really sure what my values are in relation to my work life, so I'm still not really sure how to even define Self-Care.

I am worried that if I slow down to take care of myself, everything else will fall apart.

I don't have a supportive spouse.

I am the only one making money for my family, so I couldn't possibly work fewer hours.

I have seniority at work and have the flexibility at work, so even though I hate my job, I couldn't possibly leave and find alternative employment at this stage in my life.

When creating your Self-Care Plan and considering barriers, it is also imperative that you consider your employer and your working environment. Are they supportive of your plan or are they a barrier? The research is very clear — employment conditions are directly linked to individual health. In fact, there are more reports coming out about this every day. As this is the case, employers have a responsibility to provide an environment, opportunities, and a system that supports wellness, health, and Self-Care. Where does your employer fall on this spectrum?

Take a minute to make note of any of your barriers to Self-Care in your workbook.

Take the Time to Prioritize

> *You gotta make it a priority to make your priorities a priority.*
> Richie Norton, bestselling author, international speaker, consultant

I have often found taking the time to prioritize very hard to pull off. I am interested in lots of things and I want to do everything. I have always found it difficult to prioritize one thing I love over another. I also find it hard to prioritize the *musts* and the *shoulds*. We are making decisions about our priorities all day long, even if we don't realize it. We often say, "I don't have time" when what we really mean is "I am not making that a priority." When we take the time to prioritize, it can be amazingly easy to find more time!

Here is a mid-career guidance counselor, Katrina, who is currently working at a university for an educational talent-search program providing academic advising to limited-income students in Grades 6 to 12, who will be first in their family to go to college. She was struggling with time management and seeing all her students within her work hours. This meant she was doing a lot of her preparation and paperwork at home during her "non-work" hours. This, of course, disrupts her balance, but also has the potential to lead to burnout and certainly resentment and a decrease in her ability and interest to do her work.

> *I talked with a coworker who manages her time well and I have learned and adopted her system. Instead of meeting with students individually, I am now scheduling 2–3 students at a time, which leaves extra time for me at the*

end of the day to do my prep work, instead of having to do it at home on my "off time." This strategy has worked wonders for me. This system organizes my time and my clients. This is the current biggest piece of my self-care plan where I now don't feel stressed and I am really enjoying my work.

Katrina prioritized taking the time and getting the help she needed to learn and implement a new strategy. She has prioritized her clients by using a time-management system that addresses the needs of her clients, as well as gives her more time to complete necessary paperwork. Her system also benefits the students. They get the benefit of the group and hearing each other's concerns and questions and also suggestions and support for one another. Through her ability to reach out for help and to prioritize time management, she came up with a win-win situation.

Prioritizing is HARD! Go to your workbook now and take 15 minutes to make a list of everything you do and everything you think you should be doing. This can be work stuff, life stuff, or both. That's up to you. Get it all down on paper and don't stop until you have emptied your brain of your to-do list. Next, you'll prioritize that list. Next to each item, put a "K" for keep, an "M" for modify, or an "E" for eliminate.

Go through the list once and don't think too long or hard about each item. Some will be easier than others, of course. Put the list aside and go through it again tomorrow, making any adjustments you feel you need to. All the "keepers" and "eliminators" are self-explanatory.

What about the "modifiers"?

On day number three, take your list of what you think needs to be modified and expand on it. What exactly can you do to modify each item? Perhaps you have a goal that you want to realize in the next three months, but perhaps you can modify the timeline and shoot for one year instead? Perhaps you want to get to the gym seven days a week, but modifying that goal to make it four days a week might make more sense.

We can often modify our to-dos to be a lot friendlier, without throwing our goals out the window. You may find through this process that you will want to keep or eliminate some of your modifiers. Ask yourself what you want more of and what you can let go of. Also think about how likely you are to succeed and therefore feel good about yourself and maintain your plan. If you have a goal of getting to the gym seven days a week but that is actually unrealistic and you don't make it there every day, there is a high chance you will feel like a failure and then stop going altogether.

Where Are We Now?
At this stage you have been introduced to three of the 5 Pillars of the Self-Care Revolution:
> **Pillar 1: Define Self-Care**
> **Pillar 2: Write a Values Statement**
> **Pillar 3: Make a Self-Care Plan**
>
> You have also taken action by:
> 1) Creating a working definition of Self-Care
> 2) Writing a Values Statement for yourself
> 3) Coming up with a baseline for your Self-Care Plan by stating a) what you are doing currently for Self-Care, b) what your strengths are, c) what your barriers are, and d) what your priorities are.
>
> And so ... you are ready to complete the writing of your Self-Care Plan.

Pillar 3 Making a Self-Care Plan — Post-Assessment
You will need your workbook to complete your plan.

You will use the same categories from your initial assessment: physical, spiritual, psychological, emotional, relational, professional, and environmental, as well as maintenance Self-Care and emergency Self-Care.

If you want further insight into the elements of each of these Self-Care categories, go back to the online self-assessment you completed for ideas.

Conclusion

Wow. That was a lot of work! I think so often we get good, or even great, information from so many sources. We may feel inspired, have an a-ha moment, and in general walk away from a book, movie, lecture, or conversation with some important tips and tools for change. Unfortunately, if we don't take action, and often if we don't take immediate action, those ideas and inspirations tend to fade quickly. We are back in our busy and demanding lives, and not much, if anything, changes.

I know when I read a self-help book or attend professional development training, I take *lots* of notes. Sometimes I can take notes in a handed-out packet with slides as a reference, but there usually isn't enough room for me. Sometimes I use sticky tabs and make notes in the margins of my books of my ideas and things I want to remember or do. I always need more space, and I know that I need to take action quickly if I want an idea and a plan to happen!

Your workbook serves as your action tool! At this point in the book, if you have skipped any of the assessments or exercises, I strongly encourage you to go back and complete these before moving forward.

We are moving next to "Pillar 4: Recognize Impairment and Focus on Prevention" and "Pillar 5: Support Others in Their Self-Care Plans."

Six

Pillar 4: Recognize Impairment and Focus on Prevention

Intellectuals solve problems, geniuses prevent them.
Albert Einstein, theoretical physicist

As professionals, we are responsible for being mindful of our own capacity and potential impairment. Each of our professions has some code or outline to follow, so we each have a guide we can rely on.

Pillar 4: Recognize Impairment and Focus on Prevention — Initial Assessment

You will need your workbook for this.

What is your current knowledge of professional impairment in your field? Do you have a professional organization and does it outline or define professional impairment? What does burnout look like? Do you know what compassion fatigue is and what it looks like or feels like?

Take a minute to brainstorm all that you know. Don't worry about details and don't worry about being too academic. Just jot down whatever you can think of based on your learned knowledge and based on your experience.

Think about yourself and your colleagues in the workplace. Is there a difference between burnout and compassion fatigue? If so, what do you think the difference is? What are the red flags to look out for? What other terms can you think of that define professional impairment?

Resist the urge to look anything up. This is not a quiz but a self-assessment for your own benefit. The goal will be to learn new information in this chapter that is helpful and supportive to your Self-Care. At the end, as in all of the previous chapters, you will have a post-assessment opportunity to bring it all together.

Definitions

The following definitions are from the American Institute of Stress:

Compassion fatigue: Also called "vicarious traumatization" or secondary traumatization (introduced as a concept by Figley, 1995). The emotional residue or strain of exposure to working with those suffering from the consequences of traumatic events. It differs from burn-out, but can co-exist. Compassion fatigue can occur due to exposure on one case or can be due to a "cumulative" level of trauma.

Burnout: Cumulative process marked by emotional exhaustion and withdrawal associated with increased workload and institutional stress, NOT trauma-related.

Primary traumatic stress: Primary stressors are those inherent in the extreme event, such as what was immediately experienced or witnessed, especially those things most contributing to a traumatic response.

The National Association of Social Workers, North Carolina Chapter, defines "professional impairment" this way:

> *Professional impairment occurs when something in the professional's life interferes with their ability to perform their job to the best of their ability, sometimes in a manner that can be unethical. Types of impairment include self-medicating with alcohol or drugs, maladaptive coping skills, addictions of any kind, unresolved grief, eating disorders, mental health (depression, anxiety, etc.), trauma (including vicarious), compassion fatigue, and burnout. This is not an exhaustive list.*

So, burnout and compassion fatigue and any kind of trauma are types of professional impairment. Recognizing red flags that may lead to impairment is a critical skill that all helping professionals need to hone. How can we work on this skill for ourselves and our colleagues and friends? We are generally focused on our independence and not bugging people or invading their privacy. Unfortunately this leaves us without the kind of support and accountability that preserves our Self-Care Plan, our ethical professional practice, and our sustainable prevention of burnout and impairment.

All seemed to be under control for Alice, a licensed clinical mental-health counselor with 35 years of experience. She was on top of her Self-Care and on top of making sure that others were paying attention to their own Self-Care needs, especially in the context of consistently handling stories and situations of extreme trauma. She was a critical-incident stress-management facilitator and certified trainer. If anyone was focused on Self-Care for herself and her team, she was.

> *My team was unfortunately busy with deaths by suicide and accidental deaths. We were the only such team in our state. (This is no longer the case.) I ran compassion fatigue workshops, along with skills training workshops, and also made sure that all providers at an event went through a debriefing.*

Then came September 11, 2001. This was a game-changer for her, as it was a game-changer for everyone and all our systems and basic beliefs.

> *I was called to join the Boston Trauma Team two days after September 11th, to work with a large company whose employees worked in a building at ground zero. Their building was not injured by the blasts, but because they had floor-to-ceiling windows in all directions, everyone saw the events from beginning to end.... Our job was to defuse, debrief, and provide EMDR, (eye movement desensitization reprocessing), on site if needed. Many employees were terrified to walk into the building.... The smells were powerful, the sounds of the city changed dramatically, it was quiet, the city-wide shock palpable, and the people we worked with traumatized and still in shock.*

Now remember, Alice was a seasoned mental health worker in private practice. She had a total focus on Self-Care for herself as a professional, as well as making sure that other professionals were practicing Self-Care. She did not own a TV at this time, so she had not watched the traumatic scenes played and replayed, as many had. Even though she was not at home and had access to a TV, she deliberately chose an abstinence plan to reduce any possible trauma or disturbance.

> *I worked for several days with different groups of people.... I followed my own protocols for Self-Care. I hydrated constantly, ate fresh foods, took walking breaks and engaged in other physical exercise, talked with my debriefing partner and friend, stayed in touch with my family, stayed away from the TV, and slept.*

This is a good time to go back and take a look at the plan you just created. Does your plan include any Self-Care techniques you already use on a regular basis? Are there any Self-Care techniques you use subconsciously, in light of your work and preventing trauma or burnout? Do you drink a good amount of water when you are working? Do you take breaks? Do you get outside for some fresh air? Do you have a system at your workplace of getting debriefed or debriefing others as needed? Are you getting the right amount of sleep for you and going to bed and getting up in the morning at optimal times for you and your body? You can never review your Self-Care Plan too often.

Here is more from Alice and her experience at Ground Zero shortly after 9/11:

> *What happened after I returned home I couldn't have anticipated. I began having nightmares; all the stories of the witnesses to events swirled in my head. I felt hypervigilant and felt anxiety in my body, which was not a familiar experience for me. I'm typically a pretty steady person. While* [it's] *hard to recall precisely how long this lasted, I'd say about a week. I was particularly surprised and upended by the nightmares. My sleep was impaired. I doubled my Self-Care efforts and talked with many of my colleagues, who were helpful. One colleague offered me*

> an EMDR (eye movement desensitization and reprocessing) session, which helped tremendously to re-regulate my dis-regulated body.

This experience left her with a very different understanding of how secondary trauma and secondary post-traumatic stress disorder (PTSD) could quickly affect a first responder or mental health provider, despite best efforts and understandings of Self-Care.

> I no longer take it for granted that I am well protected from the effects of another's story.

This has led Alice to implementing additional and more pointed Self-Care measures into her practice.

> I am considerably more careful about how many trauma clients I will see and how I schedule them during my day.

She attends two weekly peer consultation groups and a monthly supervision group. She believes that compassion fatigue training is an essential ingredient for mental health practitioners. Even after 35 years in practice, she finds she is impressed with the level of pain and suffering others experience, and she does not take their stories or the effects lightly.

Remember chapter two and Dylan's story about being a firefighter and the importance of Self-Care for him and his colleagues? They are really relying on science and research to help guide their prevention and Self-Care.

> Our department works with a company that offers nutritional and workout plans, along with blood tests to study the long-term effects of our job. There has been an incredible jump in participants these last ten years, with more science coming out about the dangers of life after retirement.

The work we do and the impact of that work on our bodies and minds is cumulative. We don't know when we might be impacted more significantly, as in the extreme example of 9/11, but as Alice shares, we cannot take anything for granted. The presence of a Self-Care Plan and the importance of being mindful of our potential impairments, as Dylan points out, is critical. We must be mindful every day to prevent as much negative impact as possible. We must work to preserve our wellness and thus our capacity to serve others who will need us. We must actively be on the lookout for red flags in ourselves and in our colleagues.

Although this is not an exhaustive list, here are some signs and symptoms that could indicate burnout or being on the road to burnout:

- chronic fatigue
- insomnia
- forgetfulness/impaired concentration and attention
- physical symptoms
- increased illness
- loss of appetite
- anxiety
- depression
- anger
- loss of enjoyment
- pessimism
- isolation
- detachment
- feelings of apathy and hopelessness
- increased irritability
- lack of productivity and poor performance

Helping professionals are often considered superheroes. We have to perform and be at our best and always know what to do. Often we fail to see impairment because we need to protect a professional image, ours or a colleague's. Often we are simply unwilling to consider that a colleague is not able to perform her job because of some impairment, let alone approach a colleague or report any behaviors we see.

Helping professionals are people too. We are human and we have the same rights as everyone else to ask for help when we are struggling and need support. We also have codes that obligate us to ask for help.

Don't we deserve the same care and attention that we give to the people and communities we serve?

Does your employer offer regular training in recognizing impairment, burnout, and secondary trauma? Have you had access to compassion fatigue training? Does your employer offer a safe protocol for reporting and responding to reports. This is all about trust and safety. The environment must feel safe for workers to ask for help. We must also feel safe with each other. This means our work environments need to be noncompetitive spaces. This is about collaboration and collegiality, not about competition. How do we hold each other accountable in a way that feels supportive and nurturing? How can we make sure that our employers are offering these trainings on a regular basis if they don't already? If you are self-employed, how do you find these trainings for yourself? Do you have others who are self-employed that you can collaborate with?

We will talk more about this in "Pillar 5: Supporting Others in Their Self-Care Plans."

Pillar 4: Recognize Impairment and Focus on Prevention — Post-Assessment

Here is a post-assessment that will give you tangible information about your own red flags for burnout, compassion fatigue, and professional impairment. This will give you insight into how you can prevent these in the future. Please take the time to complete this before moving on to Pillar 5. You will need your workbook.

>   Have you ever felt burned out, fatigued, or impaired?
>   If so, when, and what did it look like and feel like for you?
>   What are your own red flags that you want to pay attention to and that you want your colleagues and friends to pay attention to?
>   What do you need and want from your colleagues that would help you to prevent your own burnout, compassion fatigue, and professional impairment?

Conclusion
The goal is always prevention first, intervention second. These exist on a continuum and they are rarely linear. Self-Care exists on the same continuum. If we can't prevent something, we intervene. Following an intervention, we dive back into prevention and do our best for as long as we can.

It is my intention through this Self-Care Revolution that we live in the prevention end of the continuum as much as possible and as well as possible. This is, after all, about sustainable Self-Care. This book and these exercises are about bringing you to a place in your life and in your career where you are living your best Self-Care scenario every day, all day — by having a definition of Self-Care for yourself that matters to you and that you believe in; by having a Values Statement for yourself and your life and work that includes Self-Care; by having a written comprehensive and personal Self-Care plan; by knowing what burnout and compassion fatigue and impairment are for you and for your fellow professionals; and finally — as we will discuss in our last Pillar — by supporting others through their own personal paths of Self-Care.

SEVEN

Pillar 5: Support Others in Their Self-Care Plans

The only way we Revolutionize something is if we are all in it together.

There is an anonymously written story called "A Sense of a Goose." I love it and see it as an example of the power of supporting one another in community. Here are some of the important pieces of the story to consider as you reflect on the importance of supporting others in their Self-Care.

> *A Sense of a Goose (abridged)*
>
> *When you see geese flying along in "V" formation, and each bird flaps its wings, it creates an uplift for the bird immediately following. By flying in "V" formation, the whole flock has significantly greater flying range than if each bird flew alone. When a goose falls out of formation, it feels the drag and resistance and quickly gets back to the group in order to feel the lifting power of the bird in front. When the head goose gets tired, it rotates back in the wing and another goose flies point. Geese honk from behind to encourage those up front to keep up their speed. Finally — when a goose gets sick or is wounded and falls out of formation, two other geese fall out with that goose and follow it down to lend help and protection. They stay with the fallen goose until it is able to fly or until it dies, and only then do they launch out on their own, or with another formation, to catch up with their group.*

We can learn a lot from nature and from other animals and how well they instinctively and naturally rely on each other and other things to help them grow and be well. We can be like the geese and stick together in a formation that supports our success and wellness. What messages do you get from this story? Can we take turns doing the hardest work? If we are supporting others and getting support in return, will we be more successful at sustaining our Self-Care?

Pillar 5 Support Others in Their Self-Care Plans — Initial Assessment

You will need your workbook for this.

Are you supporting others in their Self-Care? If so, how? Brainstorm anything you can think of that you have done in the last month to support others. Have you asked a colleague how he or she is doing and encouraged any Self-Care? Have you checked in with a friend or family member who might be having an especially hard time and asked if there is any supportive thing you can do? Take a few minutes to write down any moment or incident you can recall from the last month.

Accountability

Some level of accountability always helps with follow-through. In order to write and market a successful book, I enrolled in a course. The course instructor assigned us each an "accountabili-buddy." We met once a week and had a short agenda with specific questions to ask each other. We ended the meeting by sharing our weekly goals. We also made a plan to check in mid-week via email. Once the course was over, we continued to meet. There were several course members who also continued to meet for weekly Q&A meetings with our instructor. The support, collective wisdom, and accountability were truly invaluable.

On my website, under my coaching tab, I say, "We were never meant to do this alone."

How can we formalize the supportive process a bit more with colleagues and friends? Can we write a plan down? Can we put it in our schedules to call or email or text once a week at the same time to see how the plan is going?

There is no substitute for writing down our goals with concrete plans on how to reach them. This process is a self-accountability action. There are numerous studies that point to the importance of writing down goals, and the percentage of people who reach their goals is substantially different among those who write them down. Here are some statistics to consider: 92% of people don't achieve their goals; 80% of people never set goals; of the 20% who set goals, 70% of those are not achieved; 92% of new year's resolutions fail. People with written goals are 50% more likely to achieve them, and that number increases if you share your goals with another person. (Matthews, 2015)

Secondly, there needs to be a plan for how to reach the goal. Without clear steps, there is not a clear path. At this stage, our goals become real and tangible. Hopefully they are written somewhere where we can see them easily. We have to face ourselves if we are not working toward our goals. We will be more serious and intentional about working toward and reaching our goals if we write them down and have a plan to reach them. So in addition to writing down our own Self-Care goal(s) and our plan, can we formalize a Self-Care partnership by writing down a plan for support?

Why? Why is supporting others one of the keys to the Self-Care Revolution? We do not exist in isolation. We are relational and communal beings. We thrive and succeed as others around us thrive and succeed. A Revolution cannot happen individually. We thrive on the energy, enthusiasm, and support of those around us. We are not meant to do this alone. We are meant to learn, understand, and be in relation with one another. This is how we will find our rhythm. This is how we will find and understand our own gifts, talents, and contributions. It is in relationship with others that we will learn our lessons. It is through others that we will find the support needed to be well.

I was teaching graduate school full-time for a number of years online. There were seven of us working as online faculty, dispersed throughout two countries. We would participate in weekly faculty meetings with the faculty who were on campus, and we did this at first via phone and eventually via video.

The challenges of participating in this way were many. How do you get to know one another? How do you contribute to the group? How do you feel like you are included? How do you build trust so your colleagues know and believe that you are actually working and pulling your weight? It would often take 15–30 minutes just to get the technology mostly working before the meetings could even begin.

Online faculty were at their computers early because we had to be there and be ready. As we know, in a regular live meeting people often walk in a few minutes late, or even ten minutes late. This is usually not a big deal, but if you are isolated from the group, it's harder to build trust and build relationships and build rapport, so the set of expectations is different. We barely felt we could get up to go to the bathroom or get a snack, both totally normal activities in a typical face-to-face meeting.

Because we were each other's lifelines, we would use technology as a way to support one another, in these meetings and during the week. As a colleague might walk down the hall to chat, or as colleagues might meet each other in the break room or go out for lunch, we would reach out and try to connect as best we could. We made sure that we didn't feel isolated and that we kept each other in check with regard to how much we were working.

Working online means working all the time. It is compulsive, but it was also mostly required. If one or more of us had an issue that was linked to the online portion of our job, we would reach out for support and advocacy, making sure that we weren't going it alone when asking for something from the school or university. The support we offered one another to stay well, stay grounded, stay balanced, and stay focused on the work we were doing that we loved, rather than getting caught up in the problems and the stress, was invaluable. Truly. We didn't always succeed, but we were not in it alone.

Work Environment

Supporting one another in our work environments happens in many ways and has unique challenges in a world with 24/7 access to media and technology. This is a story of a group of middle-school teachers who collaborate to support one another on a daily basis. This is what Sara, a special education teacher who is at the back-end of her career, had to share.

> *I have been working with middle school students for 15 years now, with this year being the first in 10 when I am supporting students who are more "typical" in their chronological development, interests, and emotions. It is rife with challenges as I seek to learn how to help these students grow from children into young teens in an increasingly complex culture. They face more difficult social challenges with the pressures of social media than prior to the advent of the cell phone. We are also tasked with helping them with the nuanced interactions they experience socially throughout the school day and via social media, mostly when it doesn't go smoothly and there is tension/ anger/ hurt from something that occurred online. It is a time of great transition in education, as students are allowed/ expected to use their electronics throughout their school day for educational purposes but not for social.*

Sara is speaking to another shift in our culture that has been happening for a while but has now taken hold, which is our media and technology access. Having access to media 24/7 is challenging for adults when it comes to balance and boundaries and Self-Care. Young children don't even realize the challenges, as they don't have the insight or perspective of their lives without this access to technology. We are negotiating more in our workplaces, due to the changes in our lives through technology and globalization. Sara shared that students' emotional needs at this middle-school age are the most challenging for her, particularly her students with learning disabilities. She cites Grade 7 as a perfect storm of being found out, of not fitting in, of being rejected, and of being honest to oneself and others.

> *Supporting these students takes a lot of energy on the part of the adults who teach and work with them.*

This intentional process of taking inventory of what your work entails is a critical component to understanding what you are managing and what your colleagues are also managing. Helping professionals have chosen a life of service, and that service is part of our Self-Care also. We do not often define our Self-Care by our work, but rather by how we take breaks from our difficult work. If we broaden our view of Self-Care, we have a better perspective of how we are doing. If we are living out our values, that is Self-Care. If we are doing work we are passionate about, that is Self-Care. If we have compassion for our clients and have skills and talents that can help our clients, we are practicing Self-Care. If we are doing that within the context of a work environment where our colleagues are also practicing in this manner, we have an incredible foundation to build on, if only we can recognize this.

Sara recognizes the importance of collegial and work environment support for Self-Care.

> *I have found that most of my colleagues are very mindful of the emotional health needs of both students and those of us who teach and support them. There is a camaraderie bred from sharing this chosen niche in education. For ten years, I worked in relative isolation, but switched positions and now I feel free to turn to my group for peer support. This provides an outlet for me to freely express my questions, ponderings, frustrations, worries. They in turn do the same with me. We also eat lunch together every day (teachers and paraprofessionals), and make it our intention not to talk about work at this time. We get to know each other as people separate from our teaching/supporting roles. This results in caring relationships, and carries over into our working relationships throughout the school day.*

The main thing we have control over is our own plan for Self-Care and our plan to support others. We don't always have control over our working environment, though we can sometimes decide to leave one environment for another. Not everyone has the same level of luxury in their decision making. It's important to be able to assess your situation based on trusted information. Sara was able to change positions within her school to something that was a much better fit for her Self-Care. She is clearly with a group of helping professionals who have made a commitment to one another. They have made some intentional choices about how they spend their time together while at school, and the energy around being well and supporting one another is felt in waves as it extends to the children they are supporting. This is such a great example of how we can support each other's Self-Care and create an environment where wellness is a goal.

In 2015, the Rand Corporation conducted a survey of American working conditions. The study found that nearly three-fourths of Americans report intensive or repetitive physical exertion at least a quarter of the time while on the job. And more than half report exposure to potentially dangerous working conditions. One in four American workers said they don't feel like they have enough time to do their jobs, and about half reported working during their free time in order to meet expectations. Women report having more difficulty arranging time off to take care of personal and family matters than men, as well as earning less money.

We need work environments and supervisors and policies that support wellness and support our intentions, efforts, and goals for Self-Care. This is a system-wide change effort. Individuals cannot be responsible for their own Self-Care in a vacuum. If our employer or our work environment is not set up under the umbrella of wellness, and tolerates a system that is not sustainable, we will have a hard time meeting our own Self-Care goals.

Pillar 5 Support Others in Their Self-Care Plans
— Post-Assessment

You will need your workbook for this.

We rely on each other to be well, whether we do it consciously or subconsciously. Our wellness is also directly tied to our employer and workplace. Is it set up for Self-Care? Is there a plan? Is there a system of support? We have gone through the process of defining Self-Care, developing a Values Statement that includes Self-Care, writing a Self-Care Plan, and learning to recognize impairment and focus on prevention. Now how does this all come together in a way that spells out "support for others"?

What would work in your place of employment? How about wellness and Self-Care posters in the hallways? Monthly or even weekly Self-Care training or reminder emails? Could you make use of a break room for quiet, meditation, or yoga? Do you have easy access to a gym? Flexible schedules? An accountability and support system? Flexible job descriptions and training so that you can switch off doing the hardest work? How about mandatory Self-Care requirements as part of employment? Retreats?

Take a minute to brainstorm some ideas that you might bring to the table. What would work for you and your colleagues? What would support you in the Self-Care Revolution? How can your employer be part of the Self-Care Revolution? How can you support your employer? How can you support your colleagues?

Here is some inspiration from our firefighter friend Dylan and his story of employer and collegial support:

> *My shift members and I practice yoga and work out at the firehouse. We will also use a steam room or sauna the day after a shift to rid ourselves of any toxins we may have ingested. There is a feel of camaraderie when we know we are caring for ourselves outside of the workplace.*

Write down all the ideas you can come up with right now.

Conclusion

It may seem like "supporting others" runs counter to the whole notion of *Self*-Care, but I firmly believe it is one of the Pillars in the Revolution. We are helping professionals, caring for others in our work and being of service. It is significantly more important for us to be supporting one another in this work, or we are surely on a path that is unsustainable.

Part of the Self-Care Revolution is a relational and collective process where we go beyond caring for ourselves in order to do our work, and we build our work around collective Self-Care. Can we help each other define it? Can we remind each other of our values and why we do the work we do? Can we hold each other and our employers accountable to our collective Self-Care goals?

Without everyone on board, without the support of those around you, it would be a very tall order to carry through with your own plans for Self-Care. If no one else is doing it, how would you succeed by yourself? We simply don't function that way as human beings. We are relational and we live in community. We thrive based on the support we offer and receive.

The United States is based on the idea of individualism and independence, but I believe we are missing out because of this. Let's focus on interconnectedness, shared experiences, shared values, and interdependence.

Tikkun olam is a Hebrew phrase that means "repairing the world" or "healing the world," which suggests humanity's shared responsibility to heal, repair, and transform the world. Author David Levithan introduces the concept of *tikkun olam* and this notion that we are the pieces that need to come together. This reminds me of June Jordan's words, also often attributed to Hopi Elders: "We are ones we have been waiting for."

We have the collective wisdom and compassion and love to be on this Self-Care journey together. There is no one else who is going to do this for us. This Revolution is us!

Then it hits me.

"Maybe we're the pieces," I say.

... "What?" she asks. ...

"Maybe that's it," I say gently. "With what you were talking about before. The world being broken. Maybe it isn't that we're supposed to find the pieces and put them back together. Maybe we're *the pieces."*

...

"Maybe," I say, "what we're supposed to do is come together. That's how we stop the breaking."

Tikkun olam.

  David Levithan, *Nick and Nora's Infinite Playlist*

FINAL THOUGHTS

> *Self-care is never a selfish act — it is simply good stewardship of the only gift I have, the gift I was put on earth to offer others. Anytime we can listen to true self and give the care it requires, we do it not only for ourselves, but for the many others whose lives we touch.*
> Parker J. Palmer, author, educator, activist

Helping professionals — teachers, social workers, medical professionals, mental health practitioners, first responders, clergy, coaches, leaders supporting others — are all touching many lives every day. We are professionals with a responsibility to sift through the muck and be our best selves, for our own wellness and our own satisfaction as well as for those who need us for support. We are role models. Our professional codes demand that we practice Self-Care. Helping professionals are more often than not "called to their work," and cannot hope to be their best and give their best without sustained and supported Self-Care. If we want others to be well, and that is the work we are doing, then we must also do the work to be well.

I believe that through mindfulness, compassion, and love, we can set up our Self-Care Plans and support others in their Self-Care Plans so that everyone is learning their life lessons and giving their unique gifts and talents.

This book is a guide that took you through the why, what, and how of Self-Care. The 5 Pillars of the Self-Care Revolution as I have introduced them are

Pillar 1 – Define Self-Care
Pillar 2 – Write a Values Statement
Pillar 3 – Make a Self-Care Plan
Pillar 4 – Recognize Impairment and Focus on Prevention
Pillar 5 – Support Others in Their Self-Care Plans

These Pillars are for establishing Self-Care as a permanent and important part of your everyday life and work. This book is about resilience and leadership. Take this information, use it, share it, and walk the Self-Care talk. This information and your action will help you to thrive in your life and in your work.

It's time to turn inward and turn toward each other. The world is not getting easier or safer. Our work is getting harder. The need for Self-Care in a world of dis-ease could not be more critical. It's time to mindfully embrace Self-Care as a necessary Revolution. The time for thinking about Self-Care as an act of justice is now.

What's it going to take? Remember the statistics that 92% of people don't achieve their goals, 80% of people never set goals, and you are more than 50% more likely to reach your goals if you write them down and share them with someone? How do you measure up with these numbers?

I want helping professionals to see practicing sustained Self-Care, and supporting others to do the same, as a form of justice. This is a call to action to find resilience and balance, and compassion for ourselves and for others doing this work. We need to be well and we need to be thriving in order to do good, ethical work. We cannot do our best work, be our best selves, or be ethical unless we are practicing sustained Self-Care. This has to be nonnegotiable.

In this shift, when Self-Care is Revolutionized, it means a fundamental change in our way of relating to ourselves and to one another. It means that our health care systems have to change, and our legislations and regulations have to change. If we are determined and committed to being well, to loving ourselves, and to loving one another, we change the course of action. This is a Revolution.

If you got this far in the book and you are still reading, I am going to assume you are part of the Revolution. You have taken action. Take the work you have done here and make it happen. Buy a copy for your friends and colleagues. Send them to ellenrondina.com/self-care to get a baseline sense of where they are with their Self-Care. Reach out. Join our Facebook group community, facebook.com/Sustainable-SELFCARE/. Get the support you need. We will do this together.

SELF-CARE REVOLUTION WORKBOOK

**5 Pillars
to
Prevent Burnout
and
Build Sustainable Resilience
for
Helping Professionals**

ELLEN RONDINA
Find Your Rhythm

Pillar 1: Define Self-Care

> *There's only one corner of the universe you can be certain of improving, and that's your own self.*
> Aldous Huxley, writer, philosopher, humanist, pacifist

To get a baseline for where you are with your Self-Care at this moment, before you start the following exercises, take a few minutes to complete the self-care assessment through my website, www.ellenrondina.com/self-care.

The idea that we have control only over ourselves is fundamental. I believe that we each have a responsibility to be our best self while on the planet. I also believe that I cannot be and do my best unless I am living within the framework of Self-Care. We can't improve on our Self-Care if we don't really know what the term means to us. Before getting too deep into this Pillar, I'd like you to do some brainstorming.

Take a few minutes to brainstorm what Self-Care is and means to you. Avoid the urge to look up any definitions. Keep in mind that Self-Care is personal and cultural and has the capacity to move and change with us over time, and this is just your initial assessment of what you know and think in this moment. Your definition is not set in stone and it may be quite different than you imagined in your head. Perhaps at one point you thought Self-Care was one thing, but now you think it may be something different. Let your ideas flow without judgment.

Pillar 1: Define Self-Care — Initial Assessment
Try these prompts if you don't know where to start.

Think about your five senses. What does Self-Care feel like, look like, smell like, taste like, sound like to you? What are the key themes/ideas/words that come up for you when you hear the word Self-Care? Fill in the blank: "When I do _____, I feel good." Think broadly!

1) What does Self-Care mean to you?

2) How do you define Self-Care now?

Pillar 1: Define Self-Care — Post-Assessment
Looking back through this chapter and looking at your initial assessment, would you make any changes to how you define Self-Care based on your reading or any new understandings? Take a look at the answers to your assessment questions, review the organizational and personal definitions presented, and refine your own definition here. This will be your working definition. You can change it at any time. It is never set in stone.
Self-Care to me is …

Pillar 2: Write a Values Statement

> *Values are like fingerprints. Nobody's are the same, but you leave 'em all over everything you do.*
> Elvis Presley, singer, film star

A Values Statement answers why you do what you do and for whom. Values are a compass to guide your actions and decisions. Why do you do what you do? Why do you make the decisions you make?

We will always feel out of balance and out of rhythm if what we do is different from what we believe in. The *English Oxford Dictionary* defines "values" this way: "the regard that something is held to deserve; the importance, worth, or usefulness of something" and "a person's principles or standards of behavior; one's judgment of what is important in life."

Take a minute to assess where you stand in your personal life and in your current work life. Have you ever considered what your core values are? What guides your life and your decisions, including your work? In the space you are in as you read this book and consider Self-Care at a different level, take a minute to consider the why of your life. Remember, these are just assessment exercises to get you thinking and to give you an idea of where you stand. No one else ever has to see your work here.

Finding your "why" through writing a Values Statement can be an incredibly powerful tool for how you live your life, what decisions you make, and how you feel about yourself. Therefore, it will predict how well you practice Self-Care. Your values are your why.

Pillar 2: Write a Values Statement — Initial Assessment
Start by writing a list of what you value. Don't censor yourself. This is a brainstorm. You probably won't put anything on the list that you don't inherently value, but a lengthy list doesn't mean you have to include all of them in a statement.

Here are some examples of values: ethics, excellence, diversity, inclusivity, honesty, innovation, collaboration, excitement, freedom, sustainability, fun, cleanliness, integrity, simplicity, loyalty, service, compassion, hope, and, of course, Self-Care, wellness, balance, and health.

Values

You might want to choose your top three or four values and write one statement using all of them. You might alternatively choose to write one statement for each. It's entirely up to you. Part of a sustainable Self-Care Plan is to create a Values Statement for yourself and include Self-Care in it in some capacity, or create an entire Values Statement just for Self-Care. You don't necessarily need to use the word "Self-Care." You might use "wellness" or "balance" or "health" or something along those lines that you value, where you would have to practice Self-Care in order to live that value.

How do you get from your list of values to a Values Statement? Remember that your behaviors and actions are guided by your values. What do you believe in? What do you hold to be true? A Values Statement reflects what is most important to you.

Values Statement(s)

Pillar 2: Write a Values Statement — Post-Assessment
Now that you have brainstormed your list of Values, written a first draft of one or several Value Statements, and read the whole Pillar 2 chapter, you are ready to edit and polish your final Values Statement(s). Take a look at your first version above. Does anything need to be completely changed, or does it just need a small tweak? Maybe you will leave it as is. If so, just rewrite it here. You can always come back to this and change it as needed. This is yours.

Values Statement(s)

Pillar 3: Make a Self-Care Plan

> *By Failing to Prepare, You are Preparing to Fail.*
> Benjamin Franklin, author, political theorist,
> scientist, inventor, humorist, civic activist

Take the Self-Care self-assessment first, if you haven't done so already, as it will give you a starting point, help you to identify your gaps in knowledge of your practice of Self-Care, and give you some more ideas about what you can put into your plan for it to be intentional and sustainable! By completing this assessment you will also receive your results and a bit of information as to what those results may mean.

Pillar 3: Make A Self-Care Plan — Initial Assessment
What are you currently doing for Self-Care? Do you have a specific Self-Care goal or goals? Do you have any kind of specific or regular plan? Even if you don't have a written plan or have never thought of it before, take a minute to jot down everything you can think of that you do that you would consider Self-Care in each of the labeled categories: physical, spiritual, psychological, emotional, relational, professional, and environmental, as well as maintenance Self-Care and emergency Self-Care. Remember that Self-Care is comprehensive and covers many areas of our life. Tip: I would consider financial Self-Care under both "maintenance" and "emergency." Also, there are more categories here than in the online assessment.

Take a minute first to brainstorm a goal. I would encourage you to stick to a maximum of 3 goals. You may discover that as you continue with this book and workbook, your goals will be refined.

Self-Care Goal(s)

Physical

Spiritual

Psychological

Emotional

Relational

Professional

Environmental

Maintenance

Emergency

Focus On Your Strengths
Make a list of all your strengths. Here are some prompts to help you:

What do you do well? What are your unique gifts, talents, and contributions in the world? What comes naturally? What do you know how to do? What gives you confidence? What do people compliment you for? Name three of your positive characteristics. Build on these strengths when you create your Self-Care plan. What do you enjoy? What feeds you? Where, when, and how do you thrive? This is the best place to start.

Next, think about the strengths of your surroundings. What is easily available to you? What is accessible? What is aesthetically pleasing? Where do you go that you enjoy?

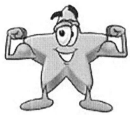

Write down as many of your strengths as you can think of.

I believe when you are operating from a strengths perspective, you are practicing Self-Care. How often are you living your strengths? How often are you functioning and working and moving through the world using these strengths? If you notice that you aren't using your strengths as often as you could, can you make any adjustments? Compare your list of strengths to the results of your Self-Care assessment. If you were practicing from more of a strengths perspective, would you be doing more things "well" in some areas that you marked as doing "okay" or "barely at all"?

Pillar 3: Make a Self-Care Plan — Identify Barriers

You will need to consider what your barriers are to practicing Self-Care. What are your barriers to Self-Care and planning for it? What are you struggling with? Why do you really believe you haven't solved the problem of not being attentive to Self-Care? What beliefs about your current situation do you know are getting in the way of moving forward? The biggest mistakes people make when they attempt to change a behavior are

    1) not identifying the barriers and, therefore,

    2) not planning on how to get over, past, or around those barriers.

    Here are some examples of barriers that other professionals have shared as they contemplated their Self-Care:

I am not a morning person and the only time I would have to myself to work out or meditate is in the morning.

I don't have the child care I need to schedule any more time for myself.

I work for an employer who doesn't value Self-Care, so the expectation is for me to never take time off.

I don't have any extra cash for any kind of Self-Care.

I'm not really sure what my values are in relation to my work life, so I'm still not really sure how to even define Self-Care.

I am worried that if I slow down to take care of myself, everything else will fall apart.

I don't have a supportive spouse.

I am the only one making money for my family, so I couldn't possibly work fewer hours.

I have seniority at work and have the flexibility at work, so even though I hate my job, I couldn't possibly leave and find alternative employment at this stage in my life.

Take a minute to make note of any of your barriers to Self-Care:

Pillar 3: Make a Self-Care Plan — Take the Time to Prioritize

Prioritizing is HARD! Take 15 minutes to make a list of everything you do and everything you think you should be doing. This can be work stuff, life stuff, or both. That's up to you. Get it all down on paper and don't stop until you have emptied your brain of your to-do list. Next, you'll prioritize that list. Next to each item, put a "K" for keep, an "M" for modify, or an "E" for eliminate. Go through the list once and don't think too long or hard about each item. Some will be easier than others, of course. Put the list aside and go through it again tomorrow, making any adjustments you feel you need to.

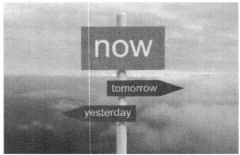

Pillar 3: Make a Self-Care Plan — Post-Assessment

This is your chance to use everything from the book and everything from what you've done in this workbook, and write out your best Self-Care Plan right now, including a revised goal. Remember that this is a living, breathing document that can be changed as necessary. No one needs to see this. This is your plan and your commitment to yourself and your wellness. You have taken a lot of action steps to get you ready for this, so use the previous exercises to help you. You will use the same categories from your initial assessment: physical, spiritual, psychological, emotional, relational, professional, and environmental, as well as maintenance Self-Care and emergency Self-Care. If you want further insight into the elements of each of these Self-Care categories, go back to the online self-assessment you completed for ideas.

Self-Care Goal(s)

Physical

Spiritual

Psychological

Emotional

Relational

Professional

Environmental

Maintenance

Emergency

Pillar 4: Recognize Impairment and Focus on Prevention

> *Intellectuals solve problems, geniuses prevent them.*
> Albert Einstein, theoretical physicist

Pillar 4: Recognize Impairment and Focus on Prevention — Initial Assessment

What is your current knowledge of professional impairment in your field? Do you have a professional organization and does it outline or define professional impairment? What does burnout look like? Do you know what compassion fatigue is and what it looks like or feels like?

Take a minute to brainstorm all that you know. Don't worry about details and don't worry about being too academic. Just jot down whatever you can think of based on your learned knowledge and based on your experience.

Think about yourself and your colleagues in the workplace. Is there a difference between burnout and compassion fatigue? If so, what do you think the difference is? What are the red flags to look out for? What other terms can you think of that define professional impairment?

Resist the urge to look anything up. This is not a quiz but a self-assessment for your own benefit. The goal will be to learn new information in this chapter that is helpful and supportive to your Self-Care.

Pillar 4: Recognize Impairment and Focus on Prevention — Post-Assessment

Here is a post-assessment that will give you tangible information about your own red flags for burnout, compassion fatigue, and professional impairment. This will give you insight into how you can prevent these in the future. Please take the time to complete this before moving on to Pillar 5.

Have you ever felt burned out, fatigued, or impaired?

If so, when, and what did it look like and feel like for you?

What are your own red flags that you want to pay attention to and that you want your colleagues and friends to pay attention to?

What do you need and want from your colleagues that would help you to prevent your own burnout, compassion fatigue, and professional impairment?

Pillar 5: Support Others in Their Self-Care Plans

We only have what we give.
Isabel Allende, author, activist

Pillar 5 Support Others in Their Self-Care Plans — Initial Assessment

The only way we Revolutionize something is if we are all in it together.

Are you supporting others in their Self-Care? If so, how? Brainstorm anything you can think of that you have done in the last month to support others. Have you asked a colleague how he or she is doing and encouraged any Self-Care? Have you checked in with a friend or family member who might be having an especially hard time and asked if there is any supportive thing you can do? Take a few minutes to write down any moment or incident you can recall from the last month.

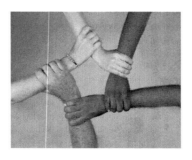

Pillar 5 Support Others in Their Self-Care Plans — Post-Assessment

We rely on each other to be well, whether we do it consciously or subconsciously. Our wellness is also directly tied to our employer and workplace. Is it set up for Self-Care? Is there a plan? Is there a system of support?

What would work in your place of employment? How about wellness and Self-Care posters in the hallways? Monthly or even weekly Self-Care training or reminder emails? Could you make use of a break room for quiet, meditation, or yoga? Do you have easy access to a gym? Flexible schedules? An accountability and support system? Flexible job descriptions and training so that you can switch off doing the hardest work? How about mandatory Self-Care requirements as part of employment? Retreats?

Take a minute to brainstorm some ideas that you might bring to the table. What would work for you and your colleagues? What would support you in the Self-Care Revolution? How can your employer be part of the Self-Care Revolution? How can you support your employer? How can you support your colleagues?

SOURCES AND ADDITIONAL RESOURCES

As my writing teachers have told me, "there are no new ideas."

There are only new ways of sharing ideas through individual experiences, stories, and perspectives.

There is a social justice theme to this book. There are theories, methods, strategies, and activities, most of which come from science and the knowledge of human behavior, change, and the brain. They are not new. I have been using this information in my coaching and teaching curriculum for well over a decade. My belief systems, opinions, the personal stories, and how I structured the book are what make this book new and hopefully effective and engaging.

As an educator and coach and someone who values ethics, collaboration, and inclusion, I honor those who have come before me. I honor the books and articles, the ideas and methods, and the theories that have guided me and have helped shape this book.

If I've told a story or collected and shared this information in a way that speaks to you and makes sense, and you take action and make important healthy changes, this book has been successful.

If you need to go elsewhere and read someone else's book to find what you need, that's great too, and you will find a list of some important books in self-care in this resources section. Please read them also. While there is a lot of overlap in self-help and self-care, there is always a new and different way of seeing and speaking about these concepts. Take what works for you, and leave the rest.

Also of note; I am not a medical doctor, nor am I a licensed psychologist. My thoughts, recommendations, and activities are not to replace sound medical and psychological evaluation and treatment.

Do your due diligence. Be critically minded. Seek out what you need.

Where to Find Ellen
Website | www.ellenrondina.com
Self-Care self-assessment | www.ellenrondina.com/self-care/
Facebook page: www.facebook.com/SustainableSELFCARE/

Quotations
Isabel Allende, author, activist | www.isabelallende.com/
Albert Einstein, theoretical physicist | www.biography.com/people/albert-einstein-9285408
Benjamin Franklin, founding father, author, inventor, civic activist, scientist, printer, politician, freemason, and diplomat | www.biography.com/people/benjamin-franklin-9301234
bell hooks, author, quote from *Communion: The Female Search for Love* | www.bellhooksinstitute.com/
Aldous Huxley, writer, philosopher | www.biography.com/people/aldous-huxley-9348198
June Jordan, poet | http://www.poetryfoundation.org/poets/june-jordan
David Levithan, author, quote from *Nick and Nora's Infinite Playlist* | www.davidlevithan.com/
Audre Lorde, writer, feminist, librarian, civil rights activist | en.wikipedia.org/wiki/Audre_Lorde
Richie Norton, author, speaker, advisor, happy guy | richienorton.com/
Sam Owens, relationship coach, author | www.relationshipscoach.co.uk/
Danzae Pace, pen name of Terri Guillemets (which is itself another pen name), writer | www.quotegarden.com/
Parker J. Palmer, award-winning author, educator, speaker, activist, founder of the Center for Courage and Renewal | www.couragerenewal.org/parker/
Elvis Presley, singer, film star | www.elvis.com/

"A Sense of a Goose" | familieslead.org/files/7614/1175/6396/Lessons_from_the_Geese.pdf

Simon Sinek, author, motivational speaker, marketing consultant | startwithwhy.com/ | www.ted.com/talks/simon_sinek_how_great_leaders_inspire_action

DaShanne Stokes, PhD, author, speaker, sociologist, social justice advocate | www.dashannestokes.com/bio.html

Other References

The American Institute of Stress | www.stress.org/americas-1-health-problem/

The American Psychological Association "Stress in America" Report | www.apa.org/news/press/releases/stress/2017/uncertainty-health-care.pdf

Bill Ervolino, staff writer, northjersey.com. "We're exhausted: Stress and social media are taking their toll." Published Oct 9, 2017 | njersy.co/2IgGvi9

Figley, C. R. "Compassion fatigue: Toward a new understanding of the costs of caring." In B. H. Stamm (Ed.), *Secondary traumatic stress: Self-care issues for clinicians, researchers, and educators* (p. 3–28). Baltimore, MD: The Sidran Press, 1995.

International Self-Care Foundation | isfglobal.org/what-is-self-care/

Susan C. Kahler. "Moral stress the top trigger in veterinarians' compassion fatigue." *Journal of the American Veterinary Medical Association.* Apr 1, 2014 (posted Dec 17, 2017) vol. 244, no. 7, p. 748–72 | www.avma.org/News/JAVMANews/Pages/150101e.aspx | doi.org/10.2460/javma.244.7.748

Gail Matthews. Research summary

Merriam-Webster defines "revolution" | www.merriam-webster.com/dictionary/revolution

My Jewish Learning. "Tikkun Olam" | www.myjewishlearning.com/article/tikkun-olam-repairing-the-world/

National Association of Social Workers, North Carolina Chapter | www.naswnc.org/

National Safety Council Survey Report | www.nsc.org/work-safety/safety-topics/fatigue/survey-report

Oxford English Dictionary defines "value" | en.oxforddictionaries.com/definition/value

The Rand Corporation 2015 Survey of American Working Conditions | www.rand.org/pubs/research_reports/RR2014.html

Self Care Forum. The Self Care Forum (UK) aims to further the reach of self-care and embed it into everyday life | www.selfcareforum.org/

Southern Poverty Law Center. The Southern Poverty Law Center is dedicated to fighting hate and bigotry and to seeking justice for the most vulnerable members of our society | www.splcenter.org/

Time magazine. "Stress, the Epidemic of the Eighties." Jun 6, 1983 | content.time.com/time/covers/0,16641,19830606,00.html

U.S. Department of Justice FBI 2016 Hate Crime Statistics | ucr.fbi.gov/hate-crime/2016/topic-pages/incidentsandoffenses

Washington Coalition of Sexual Assault Programs. The Washington Coalition of Sexual Assault Programs (WCSAP) is a nonprofit organization that strives to unite agencies engaged in the elimination of sexual violence | www.wcsap.org/

World Health Organization (WHO). "Health Education in Self-Care: Possibilities and Limitations." Report of a Scientific Consultation. Geneva, Switzerland, Nov 21–25, 1983 | www.who.int/en/

Wellness Resources that Support Self-Care
  Joshua Becker | www.becomingminimalist.com/
  Brené Brown | brenebrown.com/
  Jenny Florence | www.a-z-of-emotionalhealth.com/
  Ericka Huggins | www.erickahuggins.com/
  Barb Markway, PhD | theselfcompassionproject.com/
  Kristin Neff, PhD | self-compassion.org/
  Charlene Richard | www.charlenerichardrsw.com/
  Cheryl Richardson | www.cherylrichardson.com/
  Brianna Wiest | www.briannawiest.com/

Other Books About Self-Care for Helping Professionals
  Tim Bolen, *To the Rescue (Helping Rescue Those Who Help People)*
  Hannah Braime, *From Coping to Thriving: How to Turn Self-Care into a Way of Life*
  Tracey Cleantis, *An Invitation to Self-Care: Why Learning to Nurture Yourself Is the Key to the Life You've Always Wanted*
  Liz Garrett, *The Opposite of Burnout: 5 Career Strategies to Feel Valued, Be Heard, and Make a Difference*
  Erlene Grise-Owens (author and editor), **Justin "Jay" Miller** (editor), and **Mindy Eaves** (editor), *The A-to-Z Self-Care Handbook for Social Workers and Other Helping Professionals*
  Dan Kerrigan and Jim Moss, *Firefighter Functional Fitness: The Essential Guide to Optimal Firefighter Performance and Longevity*
  Beverly Diane Kyer, *Surviving Compassion Fatigue: Help for Those Who Help Others*
  Daniel L. Lancaster, *Burnout, Compassion Fatigue, and Vicarious Trauma: A Brief for Administrators, Physicians, and Human Service Workers*
  Alice Langholt, *A Moment for Teachers: Self-Care for Busy Teachers*
  Anana Johari Harris Parris, *Self-Care Matters: A Revolutionary's Approach*

Suzy Reading, *the self-care solution: smart habits and simple practices to allow you to flourish*

Katie Tietz, *Self Care for the Healthcare Professional: How to Gain Confidence, Take Control and Have a Balanced and Successful Career*

Melissa Wolf, MD, and Shaun Gillis, MD, *The Other Side of Burnout: Solutions for Healthcare Professionals*

Author Biography

As someone who believes that we are all responsible for supporting each other's unique gifts and talents, Ellen Rondina is a licensed master social worker (LMSW), a certified coach, a university professor, a metaphysical minister, and a professional musician. She teaches, speaks, and writes about music, wellness, spirituality, and human behavior, including self-care, mindfulness, and how to make and sustain change in one's life.

She has taught music to people of all ages, anger management to people with felony convictions, and parenting and money management to families who were experiencing homelessness. She has been sought after as a trainer and speaker in areas from bullying to mindfulness, and supported everything and everyone in between. Ellen is passionate about personal growth, discovery, spirit, and finding and helping others find their rhythm. Her mission is to guide people into their own awareness and to support them in putting their intentions into practice.

As a social justice and wellness advocate, her approach is from a strengths perspective, and she uses her broad knowledge and experience to creatively meet each person in a place that feels comfortable. She is committed to providing the space, intention, insight, and support that allows people to have empowering conversations that support self-care.

Born in the Boston, Massachusetts, area, she has had a rich journey of life experience and formal education, including growing up in a musical family and becoming a professional musician at the age of ten, traveling and studying in West Africa, and pursuing a healing path.

Ellen finds balance in her work and being with her husband and son. They love to do anything outside, especially hike and be at the beach, and their favorite family game is "Boo!"

Congratulations!

You have taken concrete action toward sustained Self-Care.

Welcome to the Revolution!
Stay connected and reach out for support. It's not a Revolution unless we are all in this together!
Website: www.ellenrondina.com
Self-Care self-assessment: www.ellenrondina.com/self-care/
Blog: www.ellenrondina.com/blog/
Contact form: www.ellenrondina.com/about/contact/
Facebook page: www.facebook.com/SustainableSELFCARE/
Facebook group: www.facebook.com/groups/SelfCareforprofessionals/

In rhythm, to your Self-Care,

Ellen

I'm Asking for a Positive Review

Positive reviews are extremely important to the success of a book on Kindle/Amazon.

If you enjoyed this book and found it useful, I'd be very grateful if you'd post an honest review.

Your support matters and makes a difference.

I read all reviews and can make changes, additions, and improvements based on your feedback.

You can leave a review in the review section on the book's Amazon page.

Click on the "write a customer review" button and you are on your way!

Thank you for your feedback and support and feel free to reach out to me directly.

Printed in Great Britain
by Amazon

Simple *Valentine* CROCHET PATTERNS

Crochet Projects for Valentine's Day

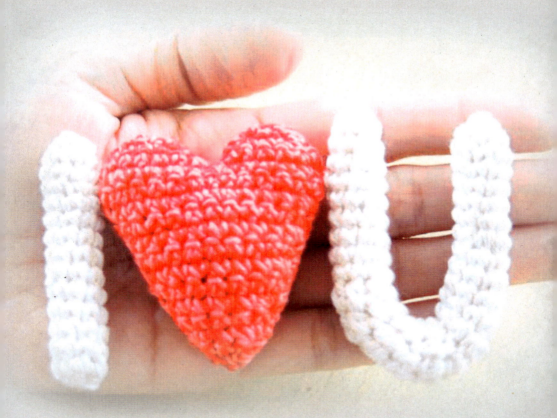